# Swim, Bike, Run–Eat

## The Complete Guide to Fueling Your Triathlon

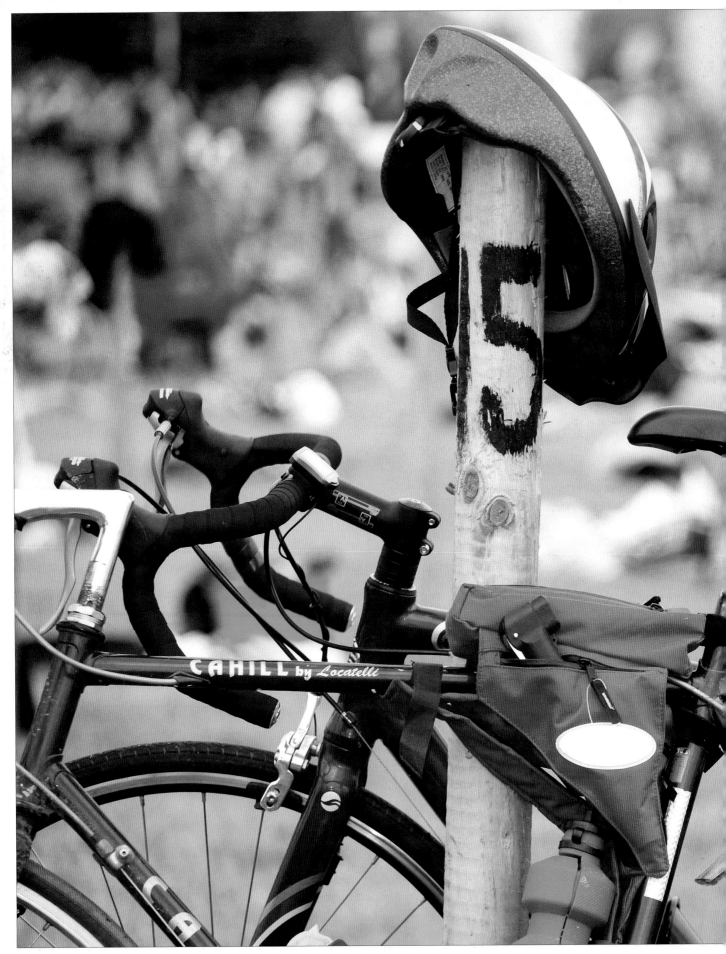

# Swim, Bike, Run–Eat

## The Complete Guide to Fueling Your Triathlon

**TOM HOLLAND,** exercise physiologist and certified sports nutritionist, and **AMY GOODSON, R.D., C.S.S.D., L.D.**

**Fair Winds Press**
100 Cummings Center, Suite 406L
Beverly, MA 01915

fairwindspress.com • bodymindbeautyhealth.com

# To Brindy

First published in the USA in 2014 by
Fair Winds Press, a member of
Quarto Publishing Group USA Inc.
100 Cummings Center, Suite 406-L
Beverly, MA 01915-6101
www.fairwindspress.com
Visit www.bodymindbeautyhealth.com. It's your personal guide
to a happy, healthy, and extraordinary life!

18 17 16 15 14        1 2 3 4 5

ISBN: 978-1-59233-606-7

Digital edition published in 2014
eISBN: 978-1-62788-023-7

Library of Congress Cataloging-in-Publication Data available

Holland, Tom, 1969-
  Swim, bike, run-- eat : the complete guide to fueling your triathlon / Tom Holland and Amy Goodson,
R.D., C.S.S.D., L.D.
      pages cm.
  Includes index.
  1. Triathlon--Training.  I. Title.
  GV1060.73.H65 2014
  796.42'57--dc23
                        2013048703

Cover design by Laura H. Couallier, Laura Herrmann Design
Book design by Laura H. Couallier, Laura Herrmann Design
Photography by Shutterstock.com: pages 10, 17, 18, 26, 28, 31, 36, 44, 52, 74, 99, 104, 110, 126, 135, 144, 168, 171, 172,
175, 176, 179, 183
Alamy: pages 2, 6, 21, 46, 73, 79, 95, 96, 114, 124, 140, 151
Getty: pages 32, 86, 60
Tom Holland: pages 14, 56, 119, 167, 186
MMRF: page 116
Revolution3: pages 123, 152
Nicole Donovan: page 132


Printed and bound in China

# Contents

**7** Foreword by Amy Goodson, R.D., C.S.S.D., L.D.

**10** Introduction

**18** PART ONE:
NUTRITION 101

**19** 1. Fuel: The Fourth Discipline of Triathlon

**26** 2. Carbohydrates

**36** 3. Protein

**44** 4. Fats

**52** 5. Hydration

**60** 6. Supplements and Ergogenic Aids

**74** PART TWO:
TRAINING FUEL

**75** 7. Dieting Down: Getting to Your Perfect Race Weight

**86** 8. Filling the Tank: Fueling Your Workouts

**96** 9. Refueling: Recovery Nutrition

**104** 10. Paleo, Vegan, All-Natural, and More: Fueling with Specialty Diets

**114** PART THREE:
RACING FUEL

**115** 11. How Do I Carry All This? Race-Day Logistics

**124** 12. Fueling Your Sprint Triathlon

**132** 13. Fueling Your Olympic Distance Triathlon

**140** 14. Fueling Your Half-Iron Distance Triathlon

**152** 15. Fueling Your Full-Iron Distance Triathlon

**168** PART FOUR:
RECIPES FOR TRIATHLETES

**169** 16. Power Meals and Power Smoothies

**184** Resources

**185** Acknowledgments

**186** About the Authors

**188** Index

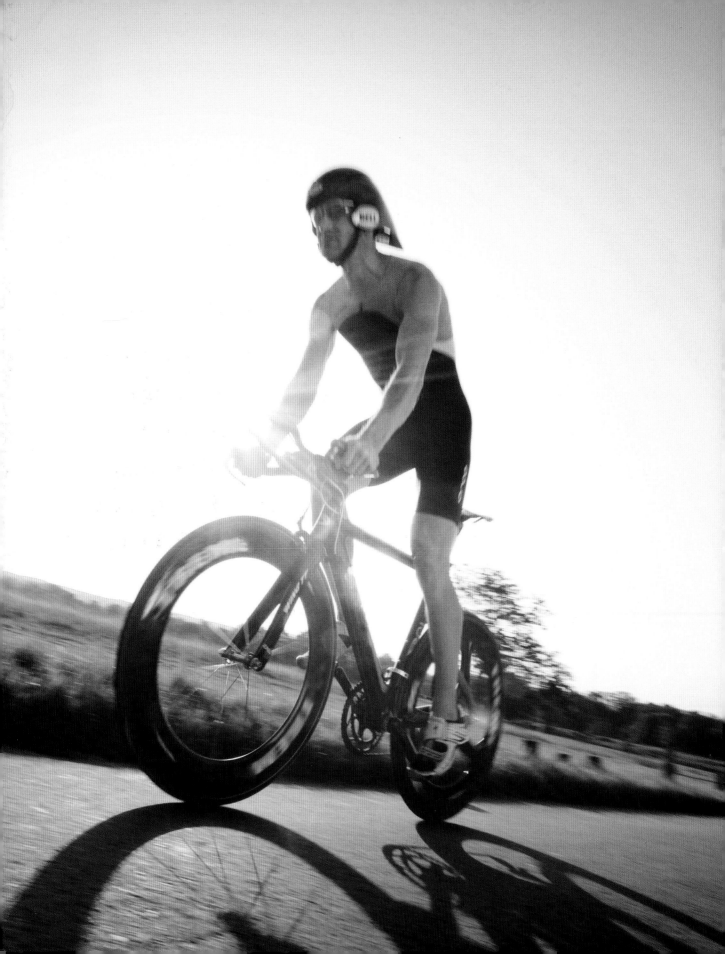

# Foreword

by Amy Goodson, R.D., C.S.S.D., L.D.

---

If you were going on a long trip, you'd fill your car up with gas, right? So when taking your body on a long trip—swimming, biking, and running—why wouldn't you fuel it up too?

One of the most common mistakes made by my triathlete clients is that they don't start thinking about nutrition until long after they begin training. Over time they realize they are always tired, they aren't recovering adequately, they aren't reaching their goals, and they can't figure out what's wrong. The answer? They forgot to put gas in their tank. No matter if the trip is long or short, it requires fuel and the better quality fuel you put in, the better performance you get out.

For most, nutrition seems daunting. It seems too difficult so they don't put much effort into it. They keep eating like they always have while they are asking for more from their bodies. The reality is nutrition is not that hard if you follow the basics and stay away from the fluff. Just because you read it in a magazine, saw it on the news, or heard about it at the gym doesn't mean it's sound science and something you should necessarily follow.

When working with clients, new to the sport or training for a full Ironman, I recommend they live by the "80/20 Rule." Eighty percent of the time, focus on eating for health and performance, fueling the body so that it works the best it can. Twenty percent of the time you can eat for pleasure, meaning that you consume foods that might be higher in calories (fat and sugar) and lower in nutrition (protein, fiber, vitamins, and minerals). In other words, sometimes you can eat what you want, but just don't eat everything you want as that can really add up. It's important to remember that every food, including chocolate cake, can be included in a healthy diet, but the key is eating more nutrient-rich foods the majority of the time and limiting the others to every now and again.

Just like you plan your training (how many hours a week you will swim, bike, and run), you should also plan your nutrition (how many meals and snacks you should eat over the course of the day). Having a game plan or a training plan will ensure that you fuel your body adequately for the trip your body is taking that day or that week. Most people who exercise regularly (i.e., those that train heavily) need to be eating a variety of meals and snacks throughout the day, including pre-, during-, and post-workout snacks. You can't wait to fuel and hydrate until your car ride to the gym because at that point it's too late. It's something you need to pay attention to from the time you wake up until the time you go to bed. Sound overwhelming? It's not if you make it a habit. Just like spending your Saturday morning biking for three hours followed by running an hour sounds pretty overwhelming to the average person, if you do it often, practice it and build up to it, it's not that hard. It becomes habit.

I'm sure you're wondering what to eat, when to eat, and how much of it to eat. Do you carb up or avoid carbs? Do you drink a sports drink during exercise or just water? Can chocolate milk actually help you recover or do you need a more traditional (i.e., gross tasting) recovery drink? That's why we're here. *Swim, Bike, Run— Eat* is designed to teach you the basics of sports nutrition and how to fuel your body, whether you are training for 30 minutes or for 5 hours and 30 minutes. If you want your car to work to the best of its ability, you give it the best fuel. You fill it up before it runs out of gas and take it for tune-ups regularly. Do the same with your body. Fuel it up with nutrient-rich fuel, hydrate it with the right liquids, and give it a tune-up each day after your training with recovery nutrition. Author Tom Holland, Ironman, trainer, and sports nutritionist and I, a sports dietitian, have years of experience working with the most elite and the most basic of triathletes. Together we have a solid base in science and can provide you with the tips, tricks, and recommendations that you need to fuel your body to perform at its most optimal level. Want to know how to be the best? Keep reading and we'll tell you how.

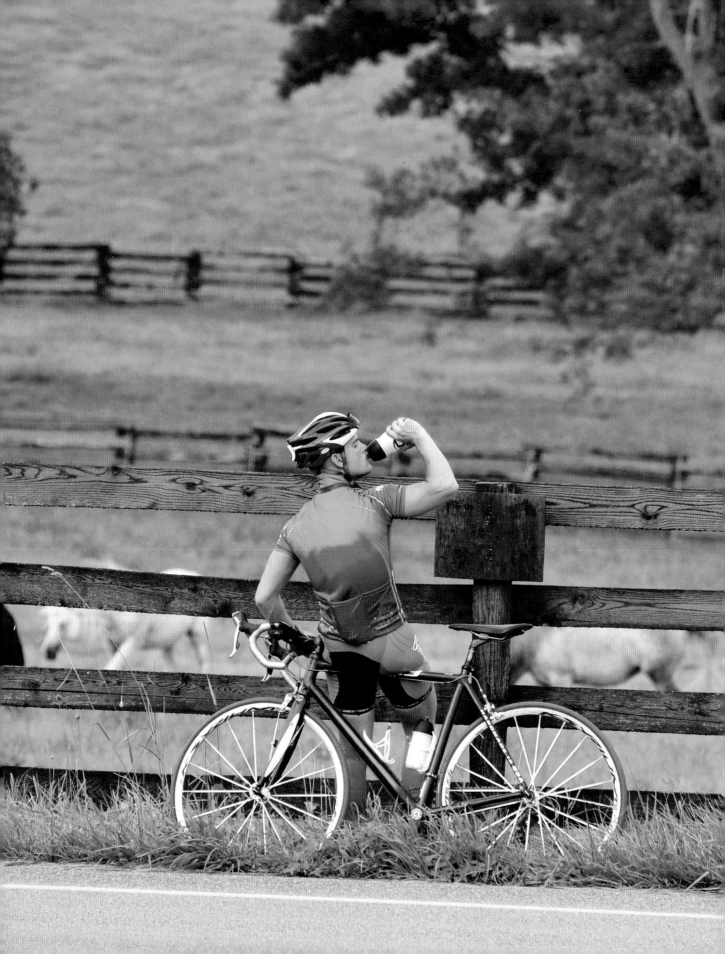

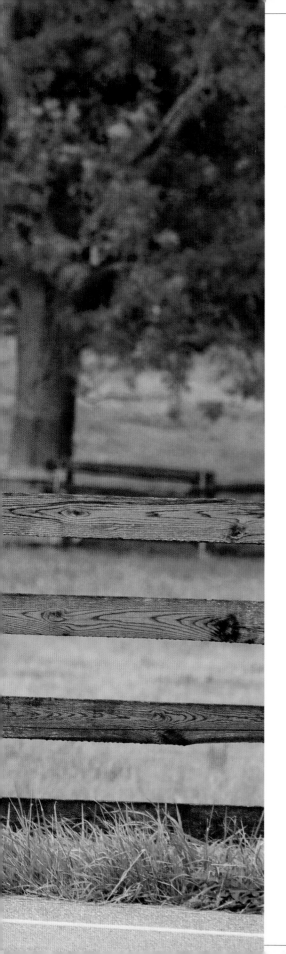

# Introduction

It was March of 1999. I was halfway around the world in beautiful Lake Taupo, New Zealand, about to take part in my first Ironman triathlon. I was a twenty-nine-year-old personal trainer who had just recently decided to make my passion my vocation, pursuing fitness as a full-time career.

Wherever you train, plan ahead for hydration and nutrition.

The decision included drastically expanding both my education as well as experience within the fitness world, going back to school to get my master's degree in exercise science and sports psychology, taking numerous other fitness certifications, and seeking out new fitness challenges.

I knew nothing about triathlons when I signed up for the Ironman; heck, I *hadn't ever owned a bike*. There were only a handful of Ironman races at the time, nowhere near the number there are today, and I certainly didn't know anyone who had ever competed in this insane 140.6-mile (226.3 km) race. But I knew I needed a huge challenge, and it would be the hardest event I had ever taken part in.

It was scheduled for March 6, the day before I was to turn thirty. The rules stated that you had to finish by midnight to be official, and my goal was to run, walk, or crawl across that line before I entered the third decade of my life. The next morning, I would wake up an Ironman.

I tend to work backward in my goal-setting strategies. I signed up for the Ironman first and then I scheduled a few short local triathlons as preparation for the full. Go big or go home. There was very little information back in the late 1990s on how to train for a triathlon, much less an Ironman. Combine this with my being a little naïve and a little cocky, and you have the perfect storm for disaster when it comes to competing in an endurance event. My training was nowhere near what it should have been, and I had no concept of fueling whatsoever.

I arrived in New Zealand a week in advance of race day. I soon became friendly with several athletes including two professionals. We were sitting at dinner a few nights before the Ironman when the conversation turned to what everyone's race-day nutritional plans. When it came my turn to answer, it went something like this:

**Pro Triathlete #1:** "So, Tom, what do you use on the bike?"

**Me:** "What do you mean?"

**Pro Triathlete #2:** "What does your bike nutrition look like? How many calories are you planning on taking in? Do you use gels, bars, or what?"

**Me:** "I have no idea what you're talking about."

The next day my newly acquired friends marched me into town and made me purchase a handful of nutritional products from a local drugstore, including a bottle of a thick, syrupy liquid that they told me was to be my main source of calories while riding the bike. (Today you would go to the expo to get these products; back then, the expos were infinitely smaller and did not offer the range of products they do today.) One pro then took me back to his room and gave me a few bottles of yet another type of strange drink, demanding that I start consuming them immediately. As I walked out, I noticed his hotel room was littered with a dozen or so empty bottles of the drink in my hands.

For my very first Ironman, I pretty much violated the two most important rules of a triathlon: I didn't train nearly enough and I had no nutritional plan whatsoever. But, thanks to my serendipitous friendship with these professional triathletes who were willing to take me under their wings and give me a last-minute fuel plan, certain disaster was averted. Their plan worked perfectly. I didn't go fast, but I never ran out of fuel. I survived the bike, ran the entire marathon, and finished with a smile on my face. Looking back and realizing how little I trained for the race, I know that the fueling plan was a huge part of my great first Ironman experience. In spite of my lackluster training and nonexistent nutrition plan, I had a great time and, when it was over, I wanted to do another.

As triathletes, we invest an enormous amount of time in our training. Unlike other sports, ours involves not just one, but three completely separate disciplines. We log thousands of yards in the pool and open water. We pedal our bikes for hours on end, sometimes while enjoying the great outdoors, other times stuck on a stationary bike. We pound the pavement, the treadmill, the trails, the track; getting our miles in for the final run. We go to the gym to lift weights. We spend month after month diligently preparing our bodies to go our respective distances.

And when it comes to triathlon, our investment of time pales in comparison to what we spend on the gear. It begins with the bike, which often costs more than our first car. We then add aero wheels and aero helmets and buy stationary bike trainers. We buy expensive GPS watches that tell us our heart rate, speed, distance, and cadence. We invest in compression socks, spandex outfits, and foam rollers.

We assemble the best machine, we purchase the best equipment, we get ourselves in the best possible shape, and then...

We completely blow it. We have no nutrition plan.

It doesn't matter how expensive our bike is or how hard we trained. If we don't fuel ourselves optimally, all of that money and all of that hard work is a waste.

What so many people fail to understand is that the nutrition plan is not just what we consume on race day. It is so much more than that. It starts long before we step foot on the starting line; it begins the very first day of training. We need to feed each and every workout. We need to refuel after each one as well.

But it's understandable that so many triathletes make this costly mistake. Let's be honest—the vast majority of people don't know how to eat properly day to day, much less how to fuel themselves while swimming, biking, and running as fast and as far as they can. There is so much confusion and misinformation when it comes to basic food and nutrition, and this can be exponentially more mind-boggling when it comes to the world of sports nutrition.

The information in this book is based on the combination of three things: my studies in exercise science and nutrition, my personal race experiences, and my experiences as a coach. I truly believe you need all three to adequately address sports nutrition. You can't just be someone with a lot of letters after your name holed up in an exercise science lab doing research; nor can you simply be someone with a long race resume who has figured out what works for you as an individual. When it comes to sports nutrition, a careful balance of the empirical and the anecdotal is

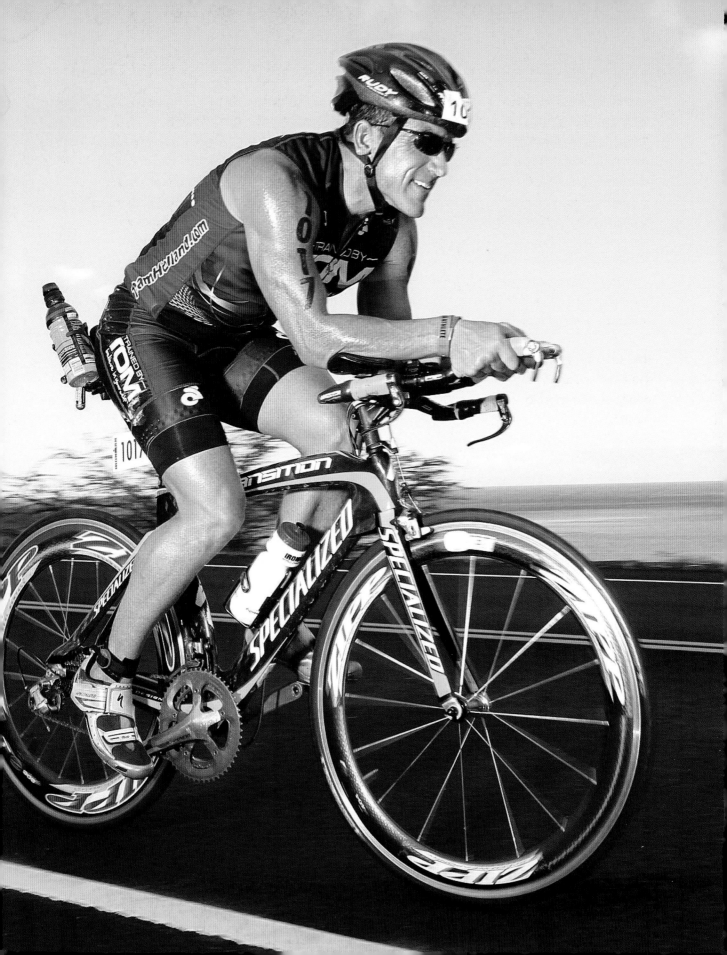

essential. What works in the controlled environment of a sports science lab often has little to no bearing on what happens out on a race course. There are simply too many variables to control.

The good news is that I personally have been your "experiment of one" for the past two decades, struggling and suffering on race courses all over the world, including Ironman triathlons in China, South Korea, Malaysia, Australia, New Zealand, Germany, and Hawaii. In addition to triathlons, I have learned how to fuel during other extreme endurance events, including the "Run to the Sun" ultramarathon, a 36-mile (57.9 km) run from sea level to the 10,000-foot (3 km) summit of Mt. Haleakala on Maui, the historic JFK 50-mile (80.5 km) race, the Rim-to-Rim-to-Rim 42-mile (67.6 km) run across the Grand Canyon and back, and 150-mile (241.4 km) bike rides from Manhattan to Montauk. Not only were many of these events all-day affairs, but also they often took place in extreme climates and at altitude that made fueling much more difficult.

In addition to my race experience, I have also been an avid student of the sport for many years. One particular group I have studied are the professional endurance athletes, paying an especially great deal of attention to those who make their living at their sport. Why? It's simple. If these people don't do well, they don't get paid. They have an enormous vested interest in performing the best they possibly can. It's their job. They can't afford not to do well. The pros are often light years ahead of the sports research because they have to be.

The goal of this book is simple. It's all about explaining in simple-to-understand terms how to fuel yourself as a triathlete—what to eat, what to drink, and what supplements to take during all phases of your training and racing. I want you to have the best race experience possible and what you eat and drink plays a huge role in both race performance and enjoyment.

But sports nutrition is a tricky thing. In sports science we are constantly searching for the elusive cause and effect when it comes to sports performance. We compare and contrast the experimental with the anecdotal. We look for patterns. We try to determine causality in our "uncontrolled experiments" known as training and racing. With the increased number and availability of training plans, in books and online, more and more people are doing the training necessary to get them to the finish line of their triathlons. We can therefore begin to look to reasons other than undertraining as the primary cause of people failing to run their best race. It's quite often not the lack of training hours that is the reason why triathletes run into problems during their races. It's the *fueling*—and lack of proper fueling before, during, and after their workouts and races.

The author biking the King K highway during the 2012 Ironman Hawaii

This book is broken up into four parts: nutrition 101, training fuel, racing fuel, and recipes. Part one explains the basics of sports nutrition and will touch on important topics all athletes should understand. It will cover the roles of carbohydrates, proteins, and fats in your diet; important information about hydration; and a primer on supplements.

Part two offers a nutrition plan to follow during training. It will explain how to get to race weight, how to properly fuel your workouts, and how to best recover post-workout. It also includes a discussion of popular diets among athletes, like the paleo and vegan diets, as well as the advantages and disadvantages of each.

Part three offers nutrition plans to follow during your race, depending on which type of race you're participating in. After covering some race-day logistics, like where to carry your racing fuel, this part discusses nutrition plans for your sprint triathlon, Olympic triathlon, half Ironman, and full Ironman.

Part four offers delicious and fortifying recipes for every athlete. These include recipes for smoothies and full meals.

If you follow the advice found in this book, I will guarantee you three things: You will look better, you will feel better, and you will go faster. It's really that simple. You just have to follow the plan.

It matters not whether you are a seasoned Ironman veteran or a "newbie" who is preparing for his or her first tri; everyone can benefit from the information found in this book. No one ever has their nutrition plan down perfectly, myself included. We must therefore constantly refine and adjust our fueling strategies as we go. What I did for my first few triathlons is vastly different from what I do today. As time passes, our bodies change, our goals change, the products change, and our fueling needs change.

When you finish reading this book, I want you to have a solid grasp of the essentials of sports nutrition. I want you to be able to pick up a gel, energy bar, or recovery drink and be able to read the label and understand what it means for you as an athlete. Is it better for day-to-day fueling, should you take it during your race, or are the ingredients perfect for post-workout recovery?

Triathlon is truly an amazing sport. It provides us with a challenging and concrete event goal to shoot for. It forces us to cross-train and to engage in three perfectly complementary sports. It gives our workouts purpose and our fitness routine a plan. It grows with us, and we can continue to participate long into our later years.

What started out for me as a crazy long-term goal in New Zealand became a life-changing event that continues to positively affect my life today. Triathlon is much more than just a sport; it's a lifestyle. I look forward to helping make your triathlon experience as special and meaningful to you as it is to me.

Proper fueling is essential to triathlon performance and enjoyment.

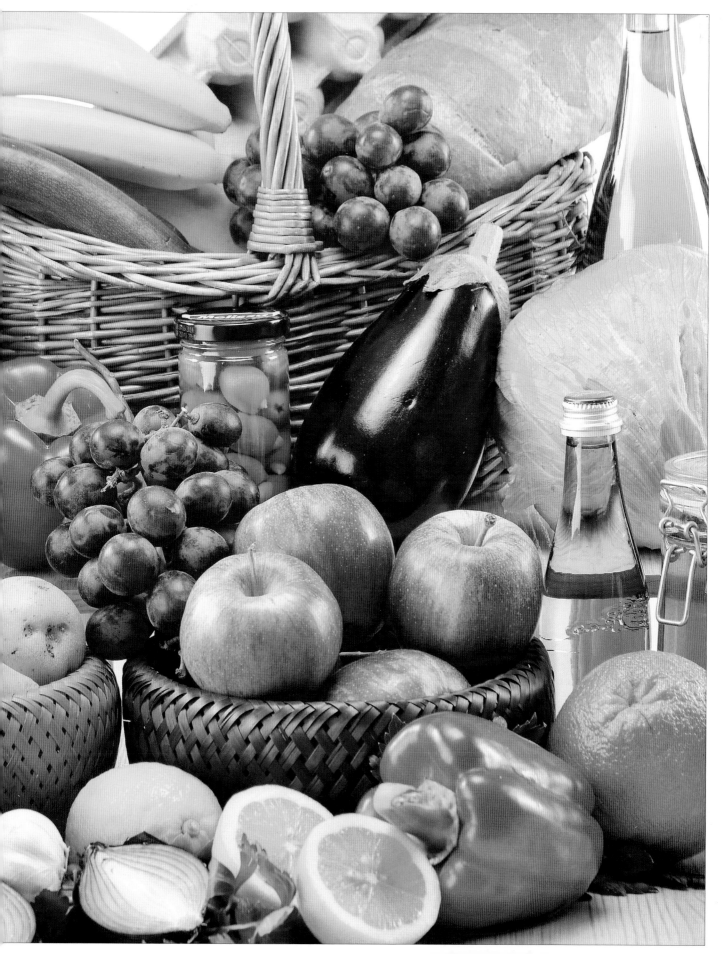

# PART 1

## Nutrition

## 101

# Fuel: The Fourth Discipline of Triathlon

**WHEN WE THINK OF TRIATHLON, WE** think of the three disciplines involved: swimming, biking, and running. These three sports are the primary focus of our training. For beginners and veterans alike, to be a better triathlete, it's pretty simple. Get in the pool and start swimming. Get on the bike and start pedaling. Lace up your shoes and start running.

What is incredible is how little time and energy is spent on what it takes to fuel these three sports—the energy itself. Energy is what endurance performance is all about. This may seem like common sense, but it bears mentioning: Food is energy. If we don't supply our bodies with the right energy in the right amounts at the right time, it matters little how much training we did. All that hard work can all go right out the window.

The different disciplines of triathlon all have their own specific fueling needs. So do the different triathlon race distances. Different climates will affect your fueling requirements as well. Different body types call for different caloric intakes. Different goals, whether your goal is to be competitive or just to finish, call for different nutritional strategies. Add to the mix individual differences in personal tastes, and you will realize how crucial it is to "dial in" your own personal triathlon nutrition plan.

Many triathletes make the mistake of only thinking about their fueling plan on race day. They fail to practice it during their workouts and don't pay any serious attention to what they eat and drink during training. Your sports nutrition plan needs to start the very first day you start training for your event. This is for several reasons, the primary being that it takes a significant amount of time to dial in what works for you. It involves constant experimentation and trial and error. Determining what exactly works for you takes time. You cannot expect to come up with your fueling plan a few days before your race and expect to perform optimally. And that's unfortunately what the vast majority of triathletes do.

**TIP:** The more time you spend on your nutrition plan before your race, the faster your time will be and the better time you will have.

It really saddens me when someone tells me about their triathlon race experience and how things went wrong, and I know from their "race report" that improper nutrition was most likely to blame. All too often the negative factors they describe could easily have been avoided with the proper nutrition plan. What's unfortunate is that they are very rarely aware that fueling was indeed the root cause of their problems, and they are therefore destined to have the same experience when they race again, unless they fix their nutrition plan.

The normal progression of triathlon is to start with the shorter distances, such as the sprint and Olympic, and then take on the longer distances over time. If you have fueling issues during your half Ironman distance race and don't resolve them before you race the full distance, the negative consequences will be magnified exponentially. The longer your race distance, the more crucial your fueling plan becomes. People tend to think I'm a little nuts when I say that doing an Ironman is not as physically hard as one might think; what makes it difficult is learning to take in the right amounts and combinations of foods and fluids to get us to the finish line. This has been my experience, and I truly believe it. Our bodies are meant to move forward, and we are physically designed to travel long distances. The main problem therefore is not the distance itself, it is ensuring that we are fueling our bodies to go the distance.

**TIP:** "DNF" means "Did Not Finish"— to quit before you reach the finish line.

I have a friend Greg who is a phenomenal athlete. We met at Ironman Lake Placid and raced there several times together. Every race started out the same: He would have a fast swim and a great bike split, but I would always end up catching him on the run. He'd be walking and in serious gastrointestinal pain, so much so that he would end up walking off the course and ultimately DNFing (Did Not Finish). He started Lake Placid four times but never once made it to the finish line. It wasn't that he didn't do the training. He definitely put in the miles. No, Greg had a major problem with his fueling. He never quite dialed in his race strategy during training, and it cost him four finisher's medals.

It comes as no surprise to me that most people don't have the slightest clue how to fuel their triathlon races and their triathlon training. Most people have a hard enough time fueling their daily lives, so how can they possibly be expected to know how to fuel three different sports, done one right after the other, often in less-than-optimal weather conditions, as fast as possible? I am constantly amazed at the lack of understanding about the very basics in human nutrition in today's society. The myths and misunderstandings when it comes to what we eat can be truly mind-boggling, especially given that this is the twenty-first century. We've been to the moon, yet millions of people still don't really know what the difference is between carbohydrates and protein.

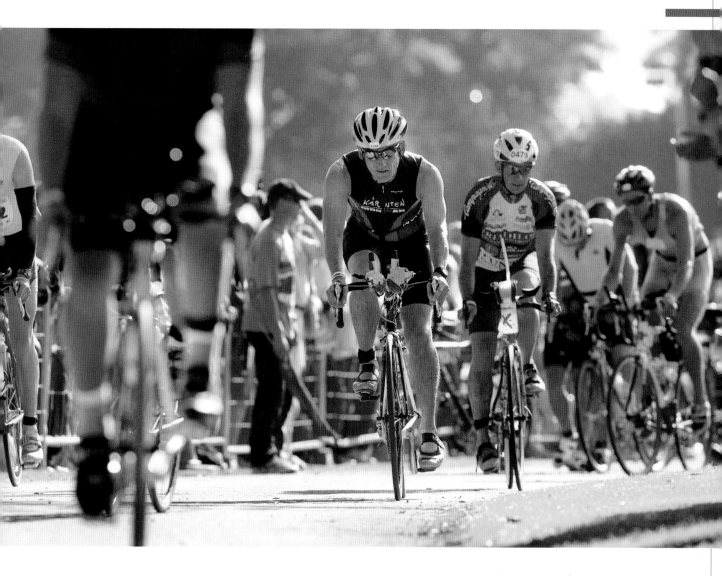

The questions about basic nutrition are numerous: What is a carb? Are carbs good or bad? How much water should I drink every day? How much protein do I need? What is a "good fat?" Is eating late at night bad for me? Isn't fruit bad for me because of the sugar? What's the best diet? Paleo? Gluten-free? Atkins?

Again, if these questions exist concerning how we can best fuel our activities of daily living, then it stands to reason that this confusion also applies to how we should best fuel our exercise, especially extreme events that can cover more than 140 miles (225.3 km) and require nine to seventeen hours of continuous movement. If we are experiencing energy crashes every day at 3 p.m. as so many do, how the heck can we be expected to swim, bike, and run for hours and hours on end without problems?

So there are the myriad questions when it comes to fueling our sports, from the recreational exerciser to the weekend warrior athlete to those wishing to push their bodies at the highest levels. What should I eat before a long workout? Do I need to take salt tablets? When should I drink during my workout? How much? How often?

## Calories

When we talk about fueling our triathlons, what we're really talking about are calories. Calories are our gasoline. They are what make our engines run. We need calories to fuel our everyday activities, and we definitely need calories to fuel our triathlons. Many of you will remember the definition of calories from grade school: It's the energy needed to raise the temperature of one gram of water one degree Celsius. So what, right? How the heck does that little nugget of information help me get to the finish line of my Olympic triathlon in a few months?

Yes, there is so much confusion today concerning the basic concept of calories. How many do we need? What percentage should be carbohydrate, protein, and fat? What's an "empty" calorie? Unfortunately, there is still so much misinformation out there as well as conflicting research; again, it's no wonder that so many people are perplexed when it comes to this subject.

Let's get back to the basics with a simple analogy, one that I will return to throughout the book. Your body is like a car, and the food you eat is the gasoline. Just as there are different grades of gasoline, from cheap to premium, there are also different grades of calories. You cannot put inexpensive fuel into a high-performance vehicle and expect it to run its best. Yet that's what so many do each and every day. They take in "empty calories," especially in the form of processed food and sugar, and thus they are fueling themselves with the cheapest, lowest-grade fuel possible. Millions of people have absolutely no idea how great they can feel if they just learned to fuel themselves with foods that supply sustained, quality energy.

The same holds true with triathlon. So many triathletes have no idea how great they could feel during training and especially during their race if they fueled themselves properly for both. People have become accustomed to depriving themselves of food, then bingeing on unhealthy food, continuing this cycle day after day, year after year. Sugar crash after sugar crash.

Most fitness professionals will tell you that getting in shape is 80 percent healthy eating. You also need to realize that, even though triathletes engage quite a bit of exercise, no amount of exercise will undo or compensate for poor eating habits. This is one of the biggest myths out there, that people who exercise can eat whatever they want. This couldn't be further from the truth.

**TIP:** EMPTY CALORIES: A food such as candy that provides little to no nutritional value

It comes down to simple math, and the math just doesn't add up. The average person will burn roughly 3,000 calories when running a marathon. Since a pound is equal to 3,500 calories, that means you are 500 calories short of losing one pound (0.5 kg) after having run 26.2 miles (42 km).

Scary, isn't it? But the math doesn't lie.

Please don't misunderstand me; exercise is a huge part of the whole puzzle when it comes to losing weight and getting in shape. When it comes to both of these concepts, one of the most common mistakes people make is that they either drastically change what they eat or drastically change how much they exercise. One or the other, neither strategy ever works in the long term. What does work are consistent small changes in both of these areas over time. The good news is that when you do in fact change both in smaller ways, it impacts your life less in comparison with drastically changing just your eating habits or your exercise alone.

A healthy weight loss goal is to lose 1 to 2 pounds (0.5 to 1 kg) per week. Most people think this is far too conservative and that weight loss goals should be much greater. So let's do the math: To lose 2 pounds (1 kg) per week translates into a seven thousand calorie deficit, or a one thousand calorie deficit per day. If you were just trying to lose the weight through exercise alone that would translate into roughly two hours of exercise performed each and every day. This is obviously extremely difficult for the average person to do, and that is why exercise alone is not the solution to weight loss.

The other side of the coin is to try to lose weight through food restriction alone. Many people try to do so using crash diets, ones that restrict entire food groups. Sure, you may see results in the short term, but unfortunately, the primary weight lost in the short term is from fluid, not fat. In addition, long-term crash dieting and food restriction typically results in lean muscle loss, which is counterproductive for athletes of any kind.

Once again, to lose just 2 pounds (1 kg) per week would mean that you have to eat one thousand calories fewer per day, every day, than you currently do. That's pretty hard for most people to do, especially on a consistent basis. I will discuss proper weight loss strategies in much greater detail in chapter 7: Dieting Down.

So the answer lies somewhere in the middle. People who are successful at losing weight and keeping it off do so with the combination of energy expenditure through exercise combined with less energy intake as a result of eating more healthful foods.

By the way, if you think losing 2 pounds (1 kg) per week is not a big deal, realize that it would translate into more than one hundred pounds (45.4 kg) lost in a year. That's pretty amazing. Lose 1 pound (0.5 kg) a week for a year? That's more than 50 pounds (22.7 kg) lost. Seem like a good strategy now?

What's pretty incredible when you start eating healthier is that you don't have to eat less food. While portion control is obviously an issue for many people, low-quality foods with empty calories are usually extremely calorically dense. Junk food packs an enormous number of calories in relatively small portion sizes. This is part of the problem with the rising obesity crisis. We think we're not eating too much simply because the portion sizes are small, when in fact, we are consuming often hundreds and hundreds of calories more than we realize. For example, grabbing a fast-food cheeseburger, though only one small food item, will provide 500 to 900 calories and typically more than thirty grams of fat based on the size of burger. You could eat one whole wheat English muffin with 1 tablespoon (16 g) of peanut butter, 6 ounces (170 g) of low-fat Greek yogurt, one banana, and a whole egg for fewer than 500 calories and less than twenty grams of fat. The healthier food choice is way more food, but way fewer calories. And they are quality calories that will appropriately fuel your body.

That's the greatest thing about eating healthy—so many of the healthiest foods such as fruits and vegetables are extremely low in calories relative to volume. So we can and should eat great amounts of them, such as big salads, large portions of lean meats, and copious amounts of vegetables. Most of the healthy food choices have far fewer calories than much smaller portions of processed and less healthy food.

## COMPENSATORY EATING

As you begin to increase your energy expenditure through almost daily swimming, biking, and running workouts, you will most likely have an increase in appetite as well. Oftentimes, it's a huge increase in hunger. This is extremely common as your body begins to adapt to the increased metabolic demands of your training. Sometimes referred to as "compensatory eating," this increase in appetite is the reason why some people actually gain weight while training for an endurance event. Just because you may be exercising more than you ever have before, this doesn't give you license to eat whatever you want. As I will discuss in chapter 9 on refueling, this increased hunger is normal and is why it is vitally important to have a proper refueling plan in place post-workout.

Fueling as it applies to triathlon can be broken down into three separate categories: pre-exercise, exercise, and post-exercise. Most people only really pay attention to fueling their exercise, and that usually just means the race itself. If you truly focus on all three components of the sports nutrition puzzle, you will not only have a great race, but you will also feel significantly better on a day-to-day basis while getting in the best shape of your life. This is why they say triathlon is a lifestyle—it forces you to make positive changes in all aspects of your life.

When I first started doing Ironman triathlons, I would be a complete mess on the weekends following my long workouts. I would often spend the rest of the day sacked out on the couch after my long Saturday brick workout and 20-mile (32.2 km) Sunday runs. Sure, part of this had to do with my being new to the distance and with my body learning to adapt to the increased stress of these workouts. After completing more than twenty Ironman triathlons and sixty marathons and ultramarathons, I now realize that a huge part of this fatigue was due to improper fueling. I wasn't fueling up adequately or correctly for these workouts, and I wasn't refueling directly afterward. No wonder I was a complete puddle after my six-hour brick workouts or three-hour runs! I started these workouts with a less than full tank, I completed them on fumes, and I failed to adequately refill my tank afterward.

As I became more knowledgeable and more experienced with my sports nutrition, I was shocked at how great I felt on the weekends after my big workouts. I no longer crashed hard every Saturday and Sunday afternoon after my workouts, oftentimes being too tired to even go out with my wife on the weekend nights. The more I dialed in my sports nutrition in all three phases, however, the better I felt all weekend long. My fatigue level was significantly less. I could continue on throughout the day almost as if I hadn't even worked out, even after hard 100-mile (161 km) bike rides and 20-mile (32.2 km) runs.

This is an extremely important point. Training for triathlon can be pretty time-consuming, especially for the half and full Ironman distances. Many of you have full-time jobs and cannot afford to stagger in to work each day completely wrecked from your training. A proper fueling plan not only translates into increased sports performance, but it also leads to increased productivity at your work as well. You will feel better all the time.

Many of you also have boyfriends and girlfriends, husbands and wives, and children, too. Triathlon can be a selfish sport if we aren't careful, and anything we can do to lessen the impact on those around us, the better. What may be surprising is that proper fueling does just that—it lessens the impact that our training has on those around us. Not only does improper fueling lead to incredible fatigue and lack of energy, but it also often leads to crankiness, irritability, and short tempers. Train too long and too hard with poor nutrition, and illness is often the result as well.

So it's really that simple. We need to focus on fueling for our triathlon so that we not only perform to our full potential during the race itself, but also perform to our fullest potential in life as boyfriends and girlfriends, husbands and wives, and fathers and mothers.

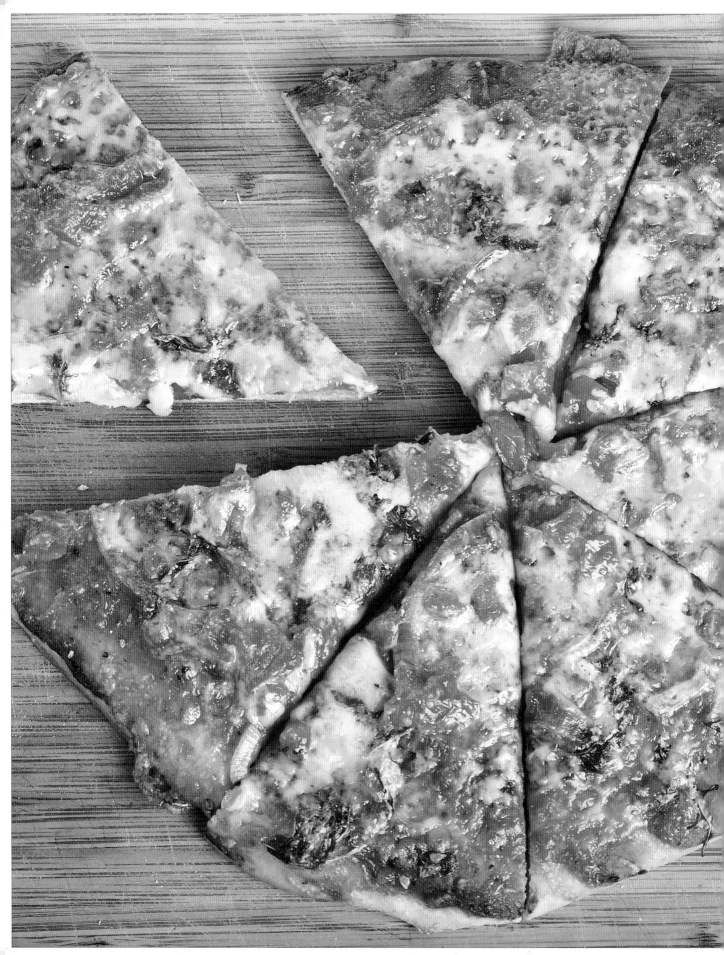

# CHAPTER 2

# Carbohydrates

**IF THERE IS ONE MACRONUTRIENT** that has received a bad rap over the past decade, it's the carbohydrate. But, like the kid in class who gets blamed for something he didn't do, the carb has been unjustly labeled. Please allow me to plead its case.

Much of this demonization has been due to the billion-dollar weight loss industry and the popularity of low-carbohydrate diets. Many believe that carbohydrates are the enemy and that they are to be avoided at all costs. This problem is compounded by the fact that these diets do often work—for the short term. Because people lose weight when they restrict their carbohydrate intake, they jump to the erroneous conclusion that all carbohydrates are indeed "bad."

It's not so.

The truth is that carbohydrates are our bodies' preferred energy source. Not fat, not protein. Carbs. Endurance athletes *need* to eat carbs to do what we do. Lots of carbs. It drives me a little crazy when someone tells me they are "off carbs." It's actually impossible to do. You simply cannot

avoid carbohydrates completely and live "carb-free." It's just not how our bodies are meant to function. This mentality illustrates both the lack of understanding about which foods actually contain carbohydrates as well as the essential role they play in our overall health and performance.

But don't sprint off to the supermarket and start loading up on cupcakes and pies just yet. Carbohydrates in and of themselves are not to be blamed for the extra pounds so many people are lugging around today. The problem lies in the *type* and *amount* of carbohydrates that people eat. Not all carbs are created equal. Yes, there are "good" carbs and there are "bad" carbs. There are complex carbohydrates and simple carbohydrates. And carbohydrates come in several forms, including sugars, starches, and fiber.

Carbohydrates are classified in three ways: as monosaccharides, disaccharides, or polysaccharides. Monosaccharides are one-unit sugars and cannot be broken down any further. Examples include glucose,

Make your homemade pizza healthier with a whole wheat crust and vegetables.

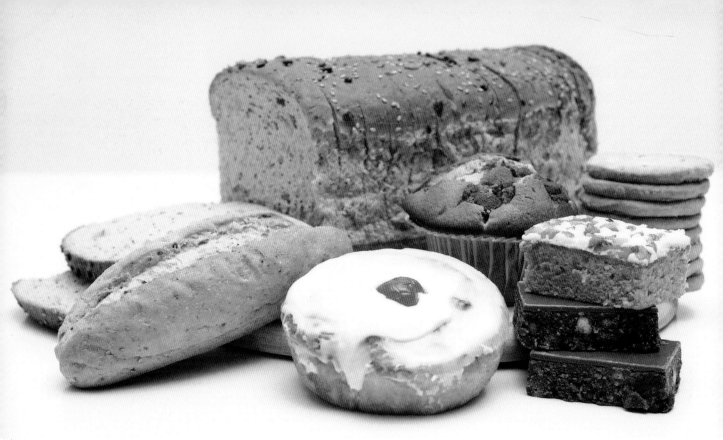

Simple carbs include cakes,
pastries, and white bread.

fructose, and galactose. Disaccharides are two monosaccharides put together, such as sucrose, maltose, and lactose. Polysaccharides are large chains of monosaccharides linked together; Glycogen is a polysaccharide and is the form in which our bodies store our carbs in our muscles and our liver. Two other polysaccharides are starch and fiber, found in plant foods. Fiber doesn't actually digest, so it works as a "bulking agent," pushing things through our gastrointestinal system and promoting good digestive health. Fiber also helps you feel full faster at meals.

Simple carbohydrates are exactly what they sound like. They are already in their simplest form, and therefore they do not require any additional breaking down. Examples of simple carbohydrates include table sugar, fructose or fruit sugar, honey, agave nectar, and corn syrup.

**TIP:** Sucrose is also known as table sugar and is a combination of glucose and fructose.

**TIP:** All carbohydrates must be broken down to monosaccharides before our bodies can use them.

Complex carbohydrates are three or more sugar chains linked together. The more chains that are linked together, the longer the body takes to break them down and release them into the bloodstream for energy as a fuel source. The kind of carbohydrate you consume is important, depending on whether you want the energy available quickly, such as during a race, or slowly, as in your daily carbohydrates fueling your everyday activities. Remember that quick fuel is followed by a rapid drop in blood sugar, which can lead to increased hunger.

Triathletes need to look at carbohydrates as our fuel. Just as we pull into a gas station before long car rides and top off our tanks, we need to do the same thing during our training and racing as triathletes. Our workouts are constantly burning carbs as our fuel, and we need to strategically fill our tanks back up. We need to do this before, during, and after our workouts as well. Just like our car, our bodies don't perform optimally if the tank is close to empty.

## THE MATH BEHIND "THE WALL"

The wall often comes down to simple math: The human body can store approximately 2,000 calories worth of carbohydrates, which roughly translates to the energy needed for twenty miles of running. Sound familiar? Most people hit the wall right around mile twenty of a marathon, exactly when their fuel tanks would be depleted without proper pre-race fueling and proper fueling during the race itself.

Again, think of your body like it's a car. It doesn't matter how fast or expensive the vehicle is, if it's not adequately fueled, it will eventually come to a loud, screeching halt, and you will be extremely unhappy when it does.

## Carbohydrates and "The Wall"

A discussion of carbohydrates is the perfect time to bring up one of the biggest enemies of the endurance athlete—the proverbial "wall." Most endurance athletes have either heard of it or, worse yet, experienced it themselves. Or perhaps you have not yet had the pleasure of hitting the wall, but you have been a spectator at the final miles of a marathon or long-distance triathlon and witnessed others experiencing this phenomenon. Also called "bonking," the wall is essentially a point during a race when the mind tells the body to keep going, but the body goes completely on strike. People experience it in different ways: lightheadedness, "dead legs," and overwhelming fatigue. The physical manifestations can vary, but the end result is always the same: You slow down, drastically. Some people slam into the wall so hard that they don't just slow down, they stop altogether. Hitting the wall is a common reason people end up having to DNF in a race.

There are two generally accepted reasons why you hit the wall: You either didn't do enough training (think long workouts) and/or you are under-fueled. I personally believe this unpleasant experience is most commonly caused by the latter, by simply running your tank down to empty.

Allow me to entertain you with a quick bonking story. It doesn't involve a triathlon, but the important lesson learned applies directly to us as endurance athletes.

One of my favorite starts to the summer is the annual Manhattan to Montauk bike ride. Taking place in May each year, it's an amazing 152-mile (244.6 km) one-day ride from the middle of New York City to the very tip of Long Island. It's relatively flat, so the course itself is not particularly challenging, but the temperature can often be a factor, so the distance and the heat can make nutrition and hydration absolutely crucial to a successful ride.

I had signed up to ride with a small group and arrived in Manhattan as the sun was just beginning to rise. As we all assembled at the start, I noticed one rider had no bike bottles, no CamelBak, no nutrition whatsoever. When I asked him what he planned on using during the ride, he said he would just eat and drink at the aid stations, which were approximately every twenty-five miles along the course.

*Not good,* I thought to myself.

## THE CENTRAL GOVERNOR THEORY

While I still believe that improper fueling is one of the primary reasons people are forced to slow down during their races, there is another theory that top sports scientists believe may be a potential cause. Known as the "Central Governor Theory," it contends that one of the reasons people slow down during an endurance event is that the brain tells the body to do so. It's a neural rather than nutritional reason. The body is being pushed to its limits, the brain recognizes this, and as a protective mechanism, it slows the body down.

**TIP:** When it comes to endurance events, a properly-fueled twenty-year-old Nissan can beat an under-fueled Ferrari every time.

This was a very long ride. It was already hot and humid at 5:15 a.m., and it was only going to get worse. To start this long journey without fueling or hydrating and to plan on only doing so at the aid stations was a recipe for disaster. Once you fall behind in your fueling, it's nearly impossible to catch up. We were going to burn thousands of calories during the ride, and if he didn't replace these calories from the very start, he would surely be in trouble.

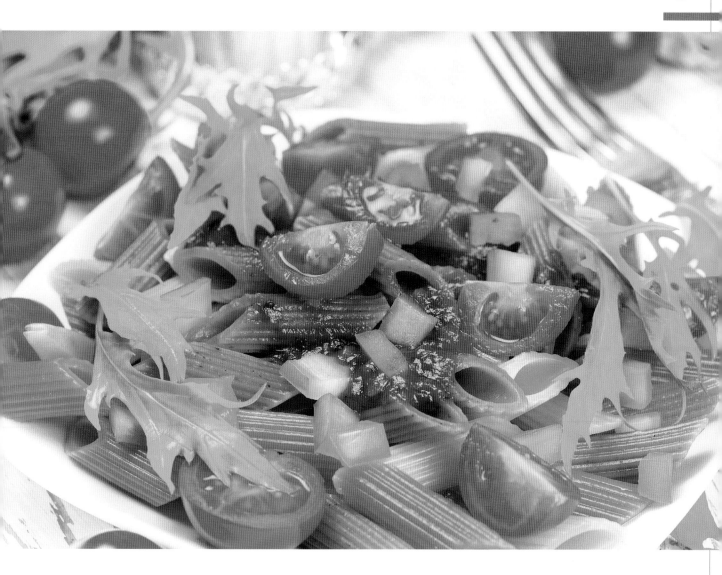

To make matters worse for him, we missed the first aid station at mile 25. So now he would have to wait until mile 50 before he would take in any real calories.

When we realized that we had unknowingly skipped the first aid station, I gave him a few sips from one of my bike bottles, which were filled with my carbohydrate and electrolyte solution. But I knew that wouldn't be close to enough. We even stopped at a convenience store along the way, where he drank a Gatorade, but I knew that wouldn't be enough, either. He needed to be taking in carbohydrates at regular intervals from mile one, not every few hours.

About four hours into the ride, he began to fall behind the group and was having trouble catching back up. He was lightheaded and starting to become disoriented. At one point, he began to turn off the course.

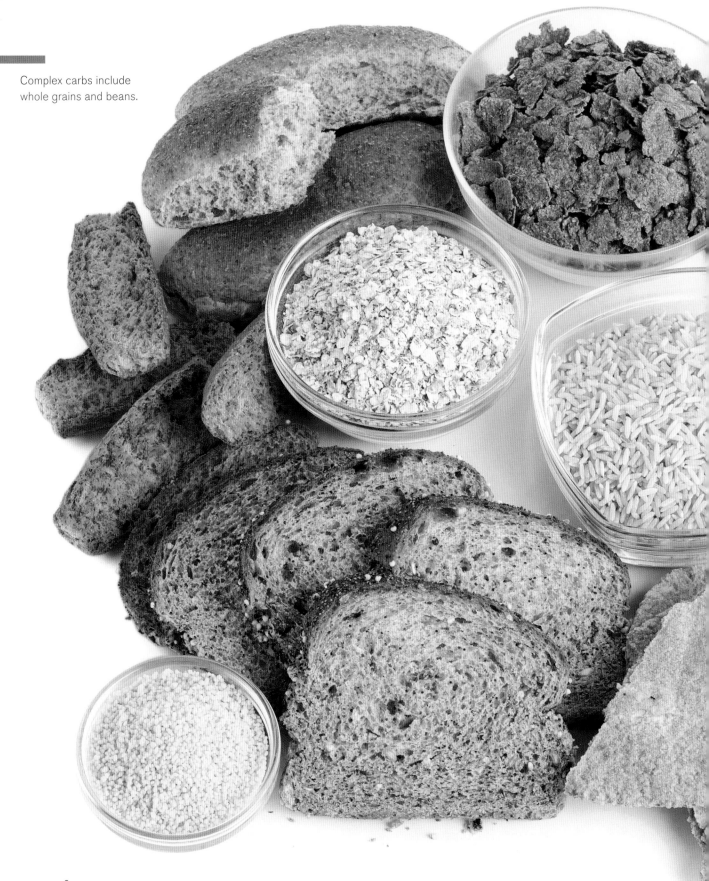

Complex carbs include
whole grains and beans.

When I asked him what he was doing, he replied that he was stopping at the aid station.

"That's not an aid station" I yelled to him, "That's a tag sale!"

His muscles and now his brain were so carb-depleted that his judgment was compromised. He was like a person lost in the desert, seeing an oasis where there was none.

Suffice it to say, he bonked and bonked hard. He had to drop off from our group and ride in on his own, creeping along at a snail's pace. He learned his lesson the hard way, that you cannot possibly start a 150-mile (244.6 km) ride with no fuel or carbohydrates and not expect to experience a bonk of epic proportions.

## Good Carbs versus Bad Carbs

We need carbs. But just what is a "good" carb and what is a "bad" carb? Most people have no idea whatsoever. This lack of understanding goes way beyond sports nutrition; it is one of the reasons we have been experiencing the dramatic rise in obesity over the past few decades. Simply put, a good carb is one that has not been refined or processed. It is relatively untouched. Examples of good carbs include whole grains, vegetables, fruits, and beans.

Good carbs are also chock full of fiber. Fiber, which is found in plant foods, cannot be digested by humans and is valuable to

**TIP:** Bad carbs: Simple, require less energy to digest. Good carbs: Complex, require more energy to digest.

us for several reasons. First, it slows down the absorption of other nutrients, which can help prevent the unwanted rise and fall of blood sugar levels. Second, foods high in fiber make you feel more satiated, which means you feel fuller, longer.

I hosted a radio show for a few years and was fortunate to interview numerous movers and shakers in the fitness industry. This included having the incredible honor of spending a full hour speaking with my idol in the world of fitness, Jack LaLanne. It all started with his being addicted to sugar as a child, and he had this simple mantra when it came to eating: "If man makes it, don't eat it."

Pretty great advice—try to eat only whole foods. The more the food has been touched by human hands, the less nutritious it usually is. Bad carbs are usually manmade. They are highly refined, stripped of their nutrients, and cause big spikes in our blood sugar levels. These spikes lead to constant hunger and the desire to eat more bad carbs. Examples of bad carbs include muffins, hamburger buns, and white rice. Other examples of simple carbohydrates include soda, cakes, cookies, chips, and alcohol.

The average adult American takes in about 20 teaspoons (80 g) of added sugar every single day according to the USDA's food consumption survey. This amounts to more than 300 extra calories per day.

The great news is that you don't have to completely give up your favorite foods. You can simply switch to a whole-grain version. You can now purchase whole-grain buns, whole-grain bread, whole-grain pasta, and whole-grain crackers.

The majority of the time, we should strive to take in carbs that are unprocessed or minimally processed whole foods. Good carbs provide the body with slow-burning energy, fiber, vitamins, and minerals. Examples of good carbs, especially for us as triathletes, include brown rice, whole-grain breads, oatmeal, and whole wheat pasta. When it comes to sugars, natural sugars such as fructose from fruit or lactose from milk are the better alternative.

Here's where it gets a little confusing. At times, athletes will want to consume bad carbs. They supply quick energy in the form of glucose, which can be beneficial during a race when we need this energy immediately. These fast-absorbing carbohydrates are also what we want to take in postworkout during the metabolic window, when our muscles are best able to absorb and restock these energy stores.

## Metabolic Window

Research has shown that there is a metabolic window or optimal time frame in which to refuel after a workout. Our bodies can best utilize both carbohydrates and protein when they are ingested within thirty minutes of exercise. The carbohydrates restock our energy supplies in our muscles and liver, and the protein helps to rebuild our muscles. The longer we wait to refuel, the less effective our bodies are at taking in these nutrients.

| THE GI SCALE | |
| --- | --- |
| High GI Foods (+70) | Sports drinks, baked potato, French fries, pretzels, and popcorn |
| Moderate GI Foods (56–70) | White rice, bananas, cola, and ice cream |
| Low GI Foods (–55) | Yogurt, milk, apples, peanuts, and grapefruit |

## The Glycemic Index

Carbohydrates can be classified in terms of their glycemic index. Originally developed to help diabetics manage their blood sugar levels, the glycemic index, or GI, measures how fast and how high a carbohydrate-containing food raises our blood glucose levels. The lower the food's GI, the less it affects our blood sugar and insulin levels.

All carbohydrates increase the blood sugar levels, but not all by the same amount. The GI scale ranges from 1 to 100, with 100 being pure glucose. Foods greater than 70 are considered high, foods 56 to 69 are considered to be moderate, and those less than 55 are considered to be low.

Ideally, pre-workout should contain low–GI foods to provide long-lasting energy to start your workout. During your workout, consume high- and some medium–GI foods because they digest quickly and thus enter your bloodstream at a faster rate. Post-workout, grab high–GI foods because they digest and are absorbed quickly, which leads to quicker recovery. Unlike typical meals during the day, a workout sugar is your friend and will help fuel and refuel you adequately.

When trying to find a high-quality carbohydrate food, look at the ratio of total carbohydrates to dietary fiber per serving, ultimately looking for one that is less than 5:1.

We as triathletes can use the glycemic index as a tool to help select the best foods for our fueling and refueling purposes. A high-fiber, or low-glycemic, food is considered one that has three grams or more of fiber per serving.

So there you have it. We as endurance athletes need our carbs to fuel our active lifestyle. We want good carbs to comprise the majority of our diet, but there is also a time when bad carbs are useful to us.

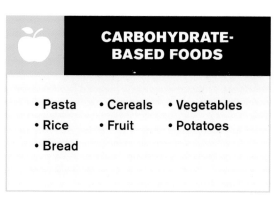

## CARBOHYDRATE-BASED FOODS

- Pasta
- Rice
- Bread
- Cereals
- Fruit
- Vegetables
- Potatoes

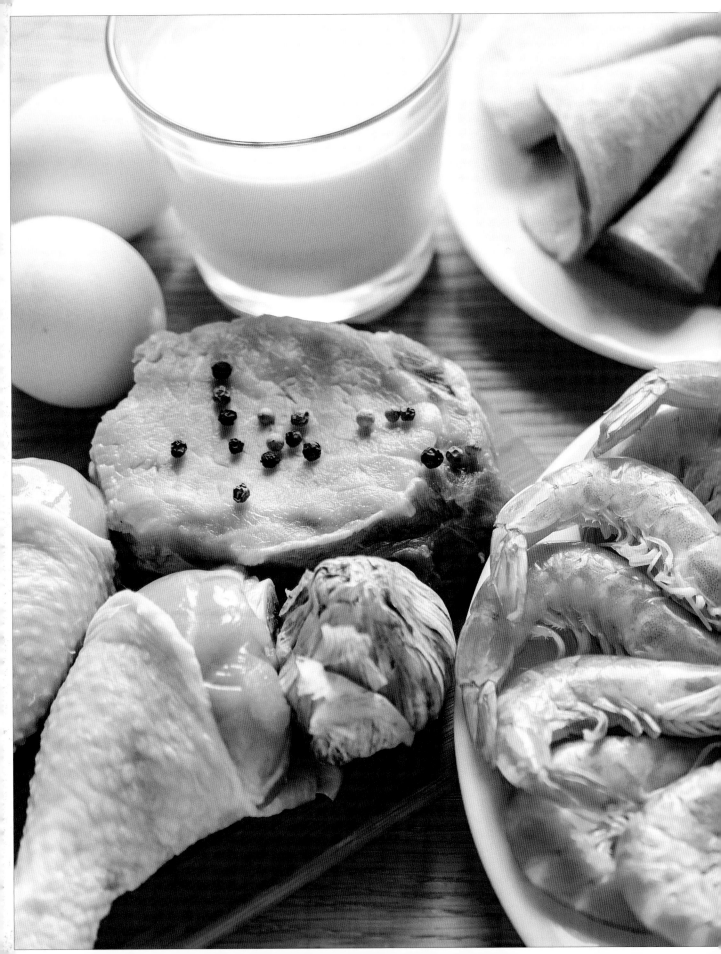

# Protein

**IF I WERE TO RANK THE MACRONUTRIENTS** in their order of importance to us as triathletes, carbohydrates would come in at a strong first place. We simply cannot live without them as our primary fuel source, to fuel both our daily lives as well as our exercise. Our muscles need carbs to get us through each and every workout and from the starting line to the finish line of our races.

Coming in a close second would be the macronutrient protein. Carbohydrates are essential in the fueling of our muscles, while protein is crucial in the building and repair of muscle tissue. Think of protein as building blocks of our muscular system. An adequate supply of protein in our diets is important in maintaining our muscular system, especially as we age.

Protein serves numerous vital functions in the body, including the formation of the brain, nervous system, and blood, and the transportation of iron, vitamins, minerals, fats, and oxygen. Protein forms enzymes that speed up reactions, they make up the antibodies that fight infections, and can be

used as energy when other fuel sources are depleted. Protein is the least "efficient" of the three macronutrients when it comes to serving as a fuel source. While our bodies do use a little protein to fuel our muscles during exercise, the contribution is extremely low relative to carbohydrates and fats. When carbohydrate stores are depleted, protein can be called upon to supply small amounts of energy; this is when the proteins in our muscle tissue can be broken down, which is not a good thing. Our goal is therefore to ensure we have adequate amounts of carbohydrate to prevent this from happening. In short, our primary goal of protein consumption is to build muscle tissue, not to fuel our muscles.

Amino acids are the building blocks of proteins. Of the twenty amino acids that form proteins, all but eight to ten can be manufactured by our bodies. Nonessential amino acids are the ones our bodies can produce on their own, and the essential amino acids are those we must obtain through diet.

Protein is essential for muscle repair and growth.

Animal sources of protein (meat, poultry, dairy, fish, and eggs) are considered complete proteins because they generally contain all of the essential amino acids. Plant-based proteins (beans, rice, grains, and vegetables) do not usually have all the essential amino acids and are therefore considered to be incomplete proteins.

**TIP:** An exception to the plant-based incomplete protein category is soy, which is in fact a complete plant-based protein.

Those who choose to avoid consuming animal protein, such as vegetarians, can solve the incomplete protein issue by combining certain plant-based proteins, which together can provide all of the essential amino acids. One example of this is the combination of rice and beans. These foods do not necessarily have to be consumed at the same meal as was previously believed to make a complete protein, but rather within a twenty-four hour time period.

I like to think of protein as my personal nutritional secret weapon when it comes to both looking and feeling good day-to-day and also for performance as a triathlete. It helps build quality lean muscle and prevent muscle breakdown after exercise. I attribute a great deal of my overall health and wellness to my focus on consuming adequate amounts of quality protein sources every day. Muscle is essential in the optimal functioning of our bodies, and protein is essential in forming and maintaining muscle.

You should strive to consume protein with every meal. This will ensure you are building new muscle tissue while also preserving the valuable muscle tissue you already have. It can be difficult for many to take in the recommended daily amount of protein each day. By spreading it out over several meals, you will find it much easier to consume protein in smaller amounts taken more frequently.

## PROTEIN SHAKES

It is always best to obtain our macronutrients from real food whenever possible. We frequently need to grab a quick meal or snack to fuel ourselves, and this is where protein supplements can be an easy way to ensure you get your daily protein requirements. There are an infinite number of protein powders to choose from, including whey, soy, egg, hemp, and more. You can use these supplements to quickly take in a large amount of protein, which is often easier than consuming the same amount with real food. There are also numerous protein bars and ready-to-drink protein shakes available for an even more convenient method of getting your protein. I personally love the FRS brand of protein drinks, a supplement line that was originally created to help cancer patients take in healthy nutrition.

Not only will consuming protein give you a healthy and strong physique by building lean muscle, but it can also help curb your appetite. Yes, studies have shown that consuming protein may add to the feeling of satiety after eating, meaning you will feel fuller longer, potentially eating less food as a result.

That's a good combination—more lean muscle and fewer calories consumed. You'll look better, weigh less, and go faster as a triathlete.

Finally, one of the additional incredible "side effects" of consuming protein and building lean muscle is the positive effect all this has on your metabolism. The more lean muscle you have, the higher your metabolic rate. Lean muscle is more metabolically active than fat tissue, which means the more of it you have, the more calories you burn twenty-four hours a day, even while at rest. Building lean muscle is pretty much the only healthy and natural way to boost your metabolism in this manner. You don't need any pills or potions with questionable results and even more questionable side effects; all you need is to exercise and eat enough quality sources of protein each day.

That's pretty darn great.

## How much protein?

There is still debate as to how much protein we need to consume daily. I believe as many others do that sedentary people generally need less protein than active people, and highly active people need even more than the average weekend warrior.

Bodybuilders and strength athletes, those for whom the goal is maximum muscular strength and maximum muscular size, tend to be at the highest end of the protein intake spectrum, often consuming one gram of protein per pound of body weight daily, oftentimes even more.

So how much is enough? I believe that the average person who exercises occasionally needs roughly one-half gram of protein per pound of body weight per day. For those who exercise more frequently and for longer durations, such as triathletes and endurance athletes, I believe that slightly more may prove beneficial, anywhere from 0.6 to 0.8 grams of protein per pound of body weight per day.

So if you are a 150-pound (68 kg) triathlete, you should shoot for anywhere from 75 to 120 grams of protein daily. You should of course modify your intake relative to the amount of exercise you do each day, consuming more protein on your longer duration workout days and days that entail multiple workouts. This becomes easy to do when you focus on your recovery nutrition, which I discuss in greater detail in chapter 9.

Realize that carbohydrates have four calories per gram, protein has four calories per gram as well, while fat has nine calories per gram. Here's some quick math on what that would look like for the following daily intakes:

**75 grams of protein × 4 calories per gram = 300 calories per day from protein**

**120 grams of protein × 4 calories per gram = 480 calories per day from protein**

## Negatives of excess protein?

There is debate as to the possible negative side effects from consuming large amounts of protein. These are the two that are commonly discussed:

Impaired Kidney Function: Some contend that excess protein intake could potentially create a strain on the kidneys and impair their normal function. While those people with preexisting kidney issues may wish to limit their protein intake, those with healthy kidneys do not seem to be at risk for adverse side effects.

Calcium Loss: While a few early studies on high protein intake demonstrated faster than normal excess calcium losses from the urine, calcium and phosphorous intake were restricted during these studies as well. Since both whole-food protein sources as well as many protein supplements contain both calcium and phosphorous, no adverse calcium content issues should accompany a high-protein diet, and a positive calcium balance may even be the result of a diet high in protein.

---

### TWO PROTEIN SOURCES TO CONSUME IN MODERATION

- **Full-fat dairy products**
- **Red meat, especially fatty cuts**

Animal products in their original form are naturally high in saturated fat, which is the type of fat that can cause inflammation and possibly lead to an increase in bad (LDL) and total cholesterol. Choosing low-fat dairy products and lean cuts of red meat reduce saturated fat per serving while maintaining the same protein and other nutrients as their high-fat counterparts.

---

### GREAT SOURCES OF PROTEIN

- **Fish, especially oily fish such as salmon**
- **Low-fat dairy products**
- **Eggs, especially those fortified with omega-3 fats**
- **Poultry**
- **Whole soy foods**
- **Beans**
- **Nuts**
- **Shellfish**
- **Wild game**

---

## Vegetarians, vegans, and protein

Even though I personally choose to eat protein from animal sources, I realize that many people, triathletes included, opt to avoid consuming meat and other animal-based protein sources. I discuss this in greater detail in chapter 10 on specialty diets. It is indeed possible to take in adequate amounts of protein from numerous alternate sources, many of which are listed on the following page. Realize that plant sources of protein are not as bioavailable in the body, thus their absorption is not as high as animal proteins. So if you are a vegetarian or vegan, you might need a little more protein so that adequate amounts are consumed and absorbed.

## Protein Values for Common Foods (Approximate)

**Fish**:

Most fish: six grams per ounce or twenty-two grams for 3½ ounces (99.2 g)

**Chicken and turkey:**

Breast: eight grams per ounce

**Beef**:

Most cuts of beef: seven grams per ounce

**Eggs and dairy:**

Egg (large): six grams

Milk (1 cup [236.6 ml]): eight grams

Cottage cheese (½ cup [115 g]): fifteen grams

Yogurt (1 cup [230 g]): eight to twelve grams (6 ounces [170 g] Greek yogurt: typically has fourteen grams of protein)

Cheese: six to ten grams per ounce

**Beans:**

Tofu (½ cup [120 g]): twenty grams

Soybeans (½ cup [86 g] cooked): fourteen grams

Soy milk (1 cup [236.6 ml]): six to ten grams

Most beans (½ cup [100 g] cooked): seven to ten grams

**Nuts and seeds:**

Peanuts (¼ cup [35 g]): nine grams

Peanut butter (2 tablespoons [32 g]): eight grams

Almonds (¼ cup [36 g]): eight grams

Pumpkin seeds (¼ cup [57 g]): eight grams

Flax seeds (¼ cup [42 g]): eight grams

Sunflower seeds (¼ cup [36 g]): six grams

Cashews (¼ cup [35 g]): five grams

It isn't easy to implement the information found in the vast majority of nutrition books. Percentages of this, milliliters of that, ounces of another—it is next to impossible to follow these types of guidelines in any consistent fashion. We are often forced to eat out at delis, restaurants, parties, and the like, where we consume food and drinks without any labels or nutritional information. How can we possibly keep track of the exact percentages of calories we consume from carbohydrates, proteins, and fats, given our lifestyles? We are not assembling our food in our kitchens for every meal, not even the majority of our meals, carefully taking food out of clearly marked containers and putting it into measuring cups or onto digital scales so that we know the exact amounts of each macronutrient and how much each contributes to our daily caloric intake. It's just not remotely possible.

So, when it comes to protein intake for triathletes, an easy starting point for how much you need each day is to divide your weight in half. Use that number as your baseline target, probably the low end, for how many grams of protein you will consume each day. It is most likely more than you are used to consuming, but if you are a triathlete and exercising frequently, this is most likely a good number for you to begin working with.

You then want to try to spread out your protein intake across the five to six smaller meals you eat each day. So if you are shooting for seventy-two grams of protein daily, and you are eating six medium-size meals per day, that's pretty simple math:

**72 grams of protein ÷ 6 meals = 12 grams of protein per meal**

Now it's obviously not always possible to get in the exact same amount of protein each and every time you eat, nor is that optimal. Sometimes you need a little more, sometimes a little less. So you may have ten grams of protein at one feeding, thirty grams at the next, twenty after a workout, and so on, finishing the day with seventy-two grams, using the example above.

Here is an example of a sample day of eating, with the protein sources in bold:

**MEAL #1:** Oatmeal with chia, **4 hard-boiled egg whites**

**MEAL #2:** Post-workout **whey protein shake** with berries

**MEAL #3:** Spinach salad with vegetables and **grilled chicken**

**MEAL #4:** Apples and bananas with **peanut butter**

**MEAL #5: Grilled salmon** with broccoli and sweet potatoes

**MEAL #6: Greek yogurt** with granola

The pattern is simple: A quality carbohydrate paired with a lean/low-fat protein source at each meal. You can choose whatever carb and protein you want, based on your personal preferences and dietary leanings; just make sure to take in high-quality sources of both at all meals. It is not possible nor is it imperative in my opinion that you always know the exact caloric value of each macronutrient. When you can determine the exact amount of protein, for example, when you are drinking a post-workout protein shake mixed with water, that's helpful. Adding up the grams of protein from egg whites is also relatively easy, as are foods such as

Greek yogurt with specific nutritional information right on their labels.

It's when you consume foods such as fish, meats, peanut butter, and other foods where you may not know the exact size and exact number of servings that determining the exact amount of protein can be challenging. My recommendation is simply to consume protein with each and every meal, regardless of whether or not you know exactly how much. That practice alone will go a very long way toward getting you down to your ideal weight, while at the same time ensuring that you are building new lean muscle and repairing the muscle you already have.

## Too much muscle?

Some triathletes waste time worrying about building too much muscle; they avoid lifting weights, and they balk at consuming adequate protein as a result, believing that they will end up looking like the guys on the cover of the muscle magazines. That's not going to happen. If your main goal as a triathlete is to go as fast as possible, then no, you don't want the physique of a bodybuilder. Having huge biceps or a huge chest will indeed slow you down to some degree. I'm also here to tell you, having been in the bodybuilding world for a short time, you will not achieve those results unless you're really trying to.

Fear of becoming too muscular is not a valid reason to avoid consuming adequate amounts of protein or even lifting weights. The type of strength routine that triathletes who want to excel at their sport should follow is vastly different from that of someone whose goal is muscular hypertrophy (growth), someone who is lifting for visual rather than performance purposes. So you need not concern yourself about taking in too much protein and becoming too muscular as a result. Those results are much more difficult than most realize, requiring extremely specific, focused, intense, and consistent workouts with heavy amounts of weight, extensive specific supplementation, and yes, often pharmaceutical interventions as well. So you need not worry about getting too "huge"—just worry about getting your protein each day.

---

**VISUALIZING GRAMS OF PROTEIN**

- **3 ounces (85 g) lean meat, chicken, or turkey** (twenty-one to twenty-four grams protein) = Deck of cards or palm of a woman's hand

- **3 ounces (85 g) fish** (eighteen to twenty-two grams protein) = Checkbook

- **1 ounce (28.4 g) cheese** (seven to ten grams protein) = Tube of lip gloss

- **2 tablespoons (32 g) peanut/ almond butter** (eight grams protein) = Golf ball

---

## Sarcopenia

Sarcopenia is a fancy scientific term for the loss of muscle we experience as we age. It is an insidious part of the aging process. After age thirty-five or thereabouts, we slowly begin to lose valuable muscle tissue each and every year. This deterioration of muscle leads to a whole host of problems, including a lowered metabolism and the subsequent weight gain, decreased strength and muscular function, and overall diminished functional ability and quality of life.

The great news is that we can in fact prevent and even reverse sarcopenia by doing two simple things as we age: First, maintaining and even building lean muscle through intelligent strength training and exercise; and second, consuming adequate amounts of protein to provide the necessary building blocks for this muscle.

So get in your protein. It's one of the three most important macronutrients in your diet. You need it in your daily diet and for refueling purposes after your workouts. Determine what specific protein sources work best for you and start making them a regular part of your daily life. You will look better, feel better, and race better as a result.

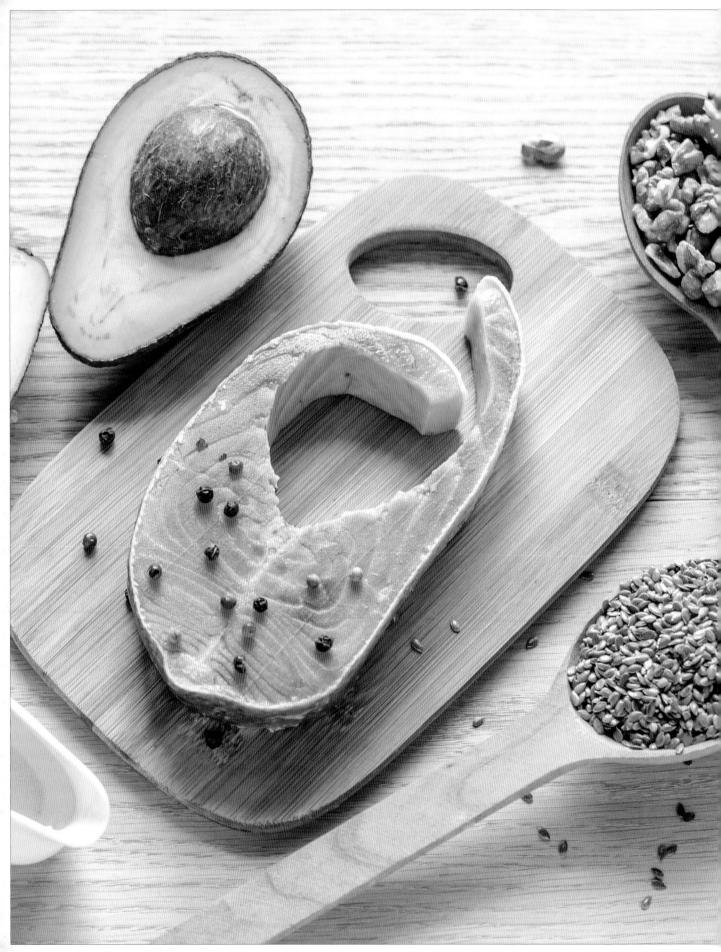

# Fats

**JUST LIKE CARBOHYDRATES AND** proteins, fats are one of the three macronutrients that can be utilized by our bodies as a fuel source. Fats contain nine calories per gram, more than double that of protein and carbohydrates, both of which contain four grams each. It seems as triathletes that we should load up our bodies with this highly concentrated source of energy, right?

Not so fast. While the human body can only store a few thousand calories worth of carbohydrates, it does in fact store tens of thousands of calories of fat. This is a confusing concept to many; if we have such great energy reserves within our bodies, how can we possibly run out during a long triathlon? Why is it necessary to take in things such as gels during the race when we have so much fat available as a fuel source?

It's a great question. The answer is that fat is simply not as efficient a fuel source as carbohydrates, especially at higher exercise intensities. We simply cannot convert fat to usable energy as quickly for our working muscles, no matter how much

we have on reserve. We use different percentages of carbohydrates and fats during different phases of exercise, and one is never the sole source of energy. We utilize more fat as a fuel source at lower exercise intensities, with the shift to the relative contribution by carbohydrates increasing as the intensity level increases.

## The skinny on fats

All fats are made up of fatty acids. They are usually linked in three-unit molecules known as triglycerides and are differentiated by their number of hydrogen atoms and their molecular bonds. Lipolysis is the process by which the body breaks down fats into glycerol and fatty acids. The fatty acids can either be broken down directly to be utilized as a fuel source, or they can be used to make glucose through a process called gluconeogenesis.

Realize that fat is not just a source of energy for the human body. It also serves a variety of other functions, including

Good fats provide a wide variety of health benefits.

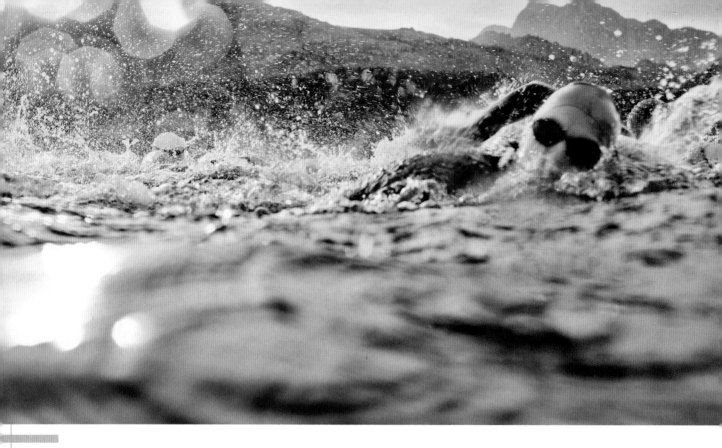

Like healthy carbs, athletes also need to make sure they take in healthy fats.

transporting vitamins A, D, E, and K, producing hormones, maintaining healthy skin, and protecting our internal organs. We need a little bit of fat in our daily diets, just not too much. Fat is a good thing for the body if you choose the right kinds of fat. Just like there are good carbs and bad carbs, fats fall into distinct categories as well.

One confusing concept for many is the fat storage process. The human body does not only store excess calories from fat as fat, it also stores excesses of any macronutrient as fat. Excesses are excesses, regardless of where they come from. So if you take in too many calories from carbohydrates, or even protein for that matter, the body will store the excess calories as fat. It all comes down to energy balance: positive and negative. Positive energy balance means you take in more calories than you expend and those calories are converted to fat, regardless of whether they are fat, carbohydrates, or protein. Negative energy balance means you burn more calories than you are taking in and thus will lose fat over time if the deficit of calories is maintained.

There are three basic types of fats found in the foods we eat:

- **Trans fat**
- **Saturated fat**
- **Unsaturated fat** (monounsaturated and polyunsaturated)

## BAD FATS

### Trans fat

The previous list is ordered from the least healthy to the healthiest types of fats. Trans fats, manmade through a process called hydrogenation, are the unhealthiest of the bunch. The chemical process involved adds hydrogen to vegetable oils to make them liquid at room temperature. Foods with trans fats last longer, are cheaper to produce, and are horrible for our health.

The myriad negative effects of trans fats include increasing our LDL (or bad) cholesterol, decreasing our HDL (or good) cholesterol, and increasing our triglyceride levels, another bad fat. Basically doing everything possible to harm our arteries and our hearts.

It is a good idea therefore to avoid eating foods containing trans fats whenever possible. There are no benefits from their consumption, and the laundry list of possible negative side effects is long and troubling. Because trans fats are found in processed foods, one of the simplest ways to avoid them is to eat whole, natural foods. Fast foods are loaded with trans fats, so, along with their relative high calorie count, which leads to weight gain, now you have two great reasons to stay away from them.

If you are reading a food label and trying to avoid this unhealthy fat, look for two things, "trans fats" and "partially hydrogenated oils." These two are both to be avoided. If you stick with foods that don't have labels such as fresh vegetables, fresh fruits, and lean cuts of meat, trans fats won't be an issue.

### TRANS FAT BAN?

As of fall 2013, the FDA has proposed to ban trans fat in foods with the goal of reducing individuals intake of trans fat to as little as possible.

### THREE FOOD CATEGORIES CONTAINING TRANS FAT

- **Stick margarine**
- **Processed foods** containing partially hydrogenated oil
- **Shortening** (such as Crisco)

### Saturated fat

The second type of fat to keep the consumption of to a minimum is saturated fat. Largely found in animal products including meats, whole milk, full-fat cheeses, and vegetable oils such as palm, palm kernel, and coconut. Saturated fats are also responsible for numerous negative health effects including increasing levels of (bad) LDL cholesterol and increasing the chances of contracting certain cancers, heart disease, type-2 diabetes, and even Alzheimer's disease.

Saturated fat also seems to wreak havoc on our appetite, affecting the hormones that regulate our feeling of fullness and satiety, possibly causing overeating as a result.

So eating some saturated fat often leads to less healthy food choices. Think of it as a saturated fat snowball effect.

As with trans fats, there are not many good things to say about saturated fats other than they taste good. While you should try to avoid trans fats whenever possible, you can keep your consumption of saturated fats to the occasional indulgence without the same health consequences. As with most things, when it comes to eating foods containing saturated fats, moderation is key. Ideally, consume 10 percent or less of total calories from saturated fat.

Here are three easy ways to keep your consumption of foods containing saturated fats in the acceptable range:

## SOME SPECIFIC FOODS CONTAINING TRANS FAT

- **Fried fast foods**
- **Chips**
- **Cakes**
- **Cookies**
- **Crackers**

When shopping, purchase the majority of your food from the outside aisles in the supermarket. This is generally where the natural, whole foods are found. Avoid the interior aisles where the food generally comes in bags and boxes, with an extensive list of ingredients, most of which you cannot pronounce and won't recognize. Finally, avoid eating at fast-food restaurants whenever possible.

**Don't overdo the butter:** Use it in moderation and/or choose butter substitutes.

**Choose low-fat dairy:** My wife has to have whole milk with her morning tea; that's nonnegotiable for her. If and when you do include dairy in your daily diet, try to choose nonfat milk and low-, reduced-, and nonfat versions whenever possible.

**Eat red meat sparingly:** Red meat is a great source of protein and other vitamins including iron, zinc, and $B_{12}$, but if you are a red meat lover, try to limit eating it to just once or twice a week. Or at least choose a lean cut of red meat such as tenderloin, sirloin, top round, or lean ground beef such as 90/10, 96/4, and 97/3 lean meat.

## GOOD FATS
### Unsaturated fats

The one good fat, of which there are two varieties, is the unsaturated kind. It includes monounsaturated and polyunsaturated fats, both of which have a whole host of positive health benefits. You should thus strive to consume foods containing these fats as part of your overall healthy eating plan.

## Monounsaturated fat

Monounsaturated fats are liquid at room temperature. They are plant-based fats and can be found in olive, peanut, and canola oils as well as avocados, nuts, and seeds. While the aforementioned bad fats impair the normal function of our arteries and our metabolisms, monounsaturated fats have the opposite effect. They can lower our levels of (bad) LDL cholesterol levels, lower our bad triglyceride levels, and possibly even raise our (good) HDL cholesterol levels. So while trans fats and saturated fats can severely harm our hearts and cardiovascular systems, monounsaturated fats can help protect and improve their function. Here are some good sources of monounsaturated fats:

- Extra virgin olive oil
- Canola oil
- Avocados
- Olives
- Hazelnuts
- Macadamia nuts
- Almonds
- Pistachios
- Cashews
- Halibut
- Mackerel
- Almond butter
- Sesame seeds
- Peanut butter
- Ready-to-eat granola

## Polyunsaturated fat

Polyunsaturated fats are also known as essential fatty acids because, just like the essential amino acids found in certain proteins, our bodies cannot manufacture them on their own. We must therefore obtain these fats though our diet.

Two of these essential polyunsaturated fatty acids are omega-3 and omega-6, also known as linolenic and linoleic acids. While omega-6 fats are common in the modern American diet, omega-3s are not. We therefore need to balance our consumption

of the two, striving to consume more foods containing the all-important omega-3s.

When it comes to omega-3s, you most likely have heard at least something about this powerful fat. Even though it seems the research on its benefits have been piling up for decades, most people have not seemed to get this message. It is still underconsumed in the typical American diet, and we therefore need to make a concerted effort to select foods containing it. These foods are good sources of omega-3s:

- Egg yolks
- Tuna
- Salmon
- Mackerel
- Cod
- Crab
- Shrimp
- Oysters
- Sardines
- Walnuts
- Wheat germ
- Flaxseeds
- Soybeans and soybean oil

You can see that omega-3s are generally found in cold-water fish, nuts, and a few plants.

Because it can be difficult to eat enough of the foods rich in omega-3s, many people, myself included, opt to take supplements containing this "super fat." Omega-3 supplements are generally taken in either liquid, capsule, or seed form. Liquid form includes products such as fish oil, which can be mixed into protein shakes for a painless way to ensure you take in this powerful macronutrient. If that doesn't work for you, swallowing a few capsules containing omega-3s can be an easy alternative. If you are purchasing a supplement, choose omega-3 supplements only because we get enough omega-6s and -9s in the diet. There is no need to supplement with the latter.

You can also get in your omega-3s by taking certain "seed supplements." As a child, my mom used to put wheat germ on our plain Cheerios, much to my dismay every morning. She was way ahead of her time nutritionally because wheat germ is known to be a good source of omega-3 fats. As I will discuss in the chapter on supplements, I continue this tradition started by my mother many decades ago, now substituting chia seeds for wheat germ on my oatmeal.

As always, I prefer to try to get as many of my nutrients from real food whenever possible. I eat large amounts of fish for this very reason, alternating between such foods as salmon, tuna, and sardines, nature's neatly packaged sources of omega-3s. Salmon is such a healthy "superfood" that I consume it at least several times per week.

The scientific studies of omega-3s are numerous, as are their reported health benefits. Hundreds of studies have been done on omega-3 consumption, and the research is promising as to the myriad of positive effects they provide. Due to this strong scientific evidence, omega-3 is one of the few supplements I personally take on a regular basis.

Here are a few of the reported positive benefits of omega-3s, a list I will reiterate in chapter 6 on supplements:

- Reduces post-workout muscle inflammation
- Lowers blood pressure
- Lowers (bad) triglyceride levels
- Improves artery health
- Reduces risk of sudden death
- Provides relief from joint pain

## The fat-burning zone

I cannot in good faith discuss fats without talking about the cardiovascular concept known as the Fat-Burning Zone. It is yet another extremely confusing concept in fitness for many to grasp, especially those who are trying to lose weight, including triathletes. I cannot count how many times I have written about this flawed topic in exercise, one that stipulates that there is greater benefit in exercising at lower rather than higher intensities because by doing so you will focus on burning fat. It's really bad exercise science and really fuzzy math.

Yes, you do in fact utilize more calories from fat as fuel at lower intensities. In fact, as you are sitting and reading this book, you are burning primarily fat calories. Big deal.

The truth is that you do not get more by doing less. The Fat-Burning Zone is flawed exercise science preached by either people who truly don't understand exercise science and the way in which the body utilizes food as fuel, and/or by people who want to lead people to believe that they can in fact avoid pushing themselves during exercise, yet reap even bigger rewards.

The truth is that while you do in fact burn a higher percentage of fat as fuel at lower intensities, you burn more total fat calories and more total calories overall at higher workloads. That's what matters when it comes to weight loss, the goal of those focused on the Fat-Burning Zone, not the relative percentage of calories burned from fat.

Put it this way: Would you rather burn 150 calories exercising at a lower intensity with 50 percent coming from fat and 75 total fat calories, or burn 200 calories while exercising for the same amount of time but at a higher intensity, with 40 percent or 80 calories coming from fat?

You burn more fat calories and more total calories by working at higher intensities. You don't get more from doing less. The people at the front of a marathon are skinnier than the ones at the back.

## HAVE SOME FAT

We as triathletes need to consume healthy fats in our diets to keep us as healthy as possible, somewhere in the ballpark of 30 percent or so of our total daily caloric intake. This is especially true for those triathletes who train frequently and eat particularly "cleanly," rarely consuming processed foods. These people can actually have a difficult time maintaining a healthy weight, and by eating the calorically dense healthy fats, they can ensure their bodies are functioning as optimally as possible.

So, to recap: Trans fats are bad, period. Saturated fats are okay in moderation. Unsaturated fats have numerous positive health benefits and are an important part of our healthy diet.

As triathletes, we want to fuel our races and our lives as optimally as possible. To do this, we need to eat a balanced diet consisting of healthy carbohydrates, healthy fats, and lean sources of proteins. There are in fact good and bad versions of all three, and we cannot consume any of them in excess. We need to choose the best versions of all three macronutrients as often as possible, consuming them in the proper percentages and in the optimal quantities.

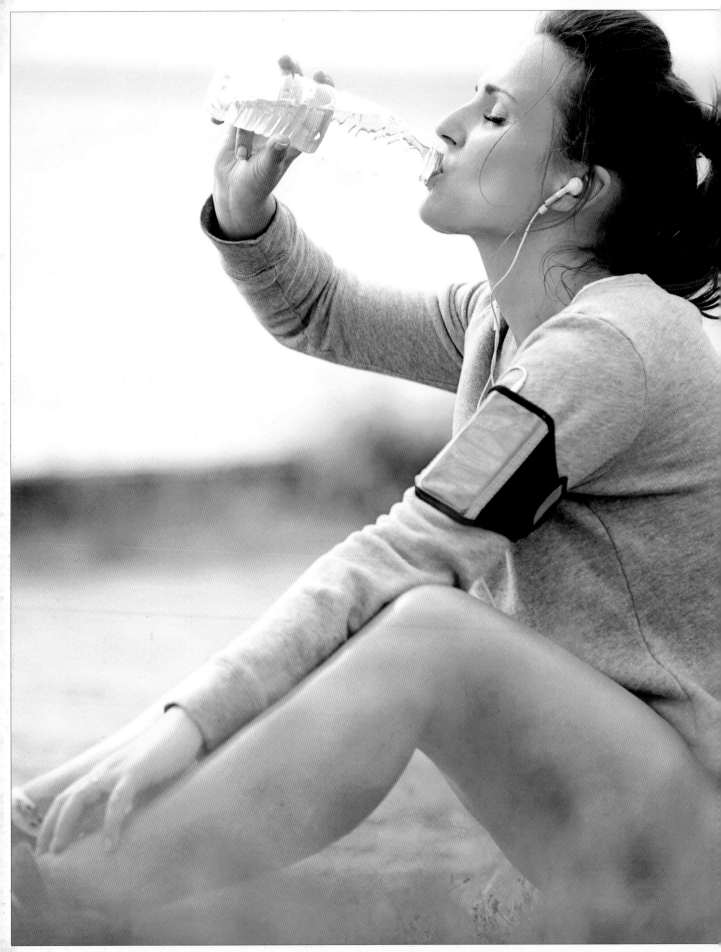

# Hydration

**OUR BODIES ARE COMPOSED OF MORE** than 50 percent water, which has a variety of functions, including temperature regulation, transporting nutrients to the cells, elimination of waste products, joint lubrication, and aiding in digestion, to name but a few. Hydration is essential to the body. We can go for a long time without food; we can only live for a short time without water.

The human body is actually one of the best machines at cooling itself down, through the processes of sweating and evaporation. We are actually better at regulating our temperature than horses, deer, dogs, and most other animals, all of whom have relatively inefficient means of cooling down during exercise. The human sweating process is however a double-edged sword when it comes to exercise. It allows us to go long distances at relatively high rates of speed, but if we don't replace what is lost in the cooling process, problems will occur.

Even mild dehydration can dramatically affect your performance

As triathletes, we sweat. Constantly. When we lose this essential water through perspiration without having it replenished, essential bodily functions are compromised. Some researchers contend that even a 2 percent loss of body weight in fluid can significantly impact our functioning. Even a 2 percent dehydration level equates to an approximate 10 percent decrease in performance. For a 150-pound (68 kg) man, this would mean that just a 3-pound (1.4 kg) loss of water weight could significantly impact his performance. And losing 3 pounds (1.4 kg) while exercising on a hot day is not difficult to do.

You often hear that we don't need to drink a significant amount of fluid because we take in water when we consume vegetables, fruits, and leafy greens. It's true that many of these healthy foods contain water, and we do get fluid as a result of eating them. But the vast majority of people are not taking in these foods on a regular basis or in significant quantities. Though a solid diet can supplement hydration, it's imperative for proper hydration that you evaluate your liquid diet.

When our bodies are dehydrated, they fail to function optimally. This can impair our regular day-to-day activities and significantly impact our bodies during prolonged exercise. Chronic dehydration can present itself in the form of fatigue and headaches in our daily lives, and during intense exercise, it can dramatically affect our performance. In cases of extreme dehydration during exercise, more dramatic problems can occur, including central nervous system issues and altered mental acuity.

## Daily hydration

Exactly how much water should we drink every day? If you have researched this topic at all, you may have seen that the advice can be all over the place. While recommendations vary widely, a simple formula you can use is to divide your weight in half and that is how many ounces of water you should be drinking daily. So if you are a 140-pound (63.5 kg) woman, you should try to consume roughly 70 ounces (2 L) of water each day. Since the vast majority of people don't really know what a pint or a liter is, seventy ounces is roughly a six-pack's worth of water. This recommendation is considerably more fluid than most people actually consume on a daily basis, which is why many health professionals believe most people are in a constant state of dehydration.

I try to start and end my day with water whenever possible. I drink a glass of water first thing in the morning when I wake up and drink another glass right before I go to bed. I purchase a liter bottle of water and try to drink from it throughout the day, refilling it when necessary. I personally have found my own hydration to be surprisingly difficult, given that it is a pretty simple practice. Since I exercise frequently and sweat liberally when I do, I am constantly trying to stay on top of my hydration. Like everything else, it comes down to preparation. I have found the best success when I keep two bottles in the refrigerator with the goal of consuming them both by the end of the day. This strategy allows me to know exactly how much I consumed and gives me an easy way to track my intake without having to guesstimate.

## URINE COLOR

There is often confusion about the color our urine should be if we are properly hydrated. Years ago, we were told that we were properly hydrated when our urine was clear. The current guidelines state that we are properly hydrated when our urine has a slight lemonade-like color. In general, avoid the extremes; we don't want our urine to be too dark or too light. A little bit yellow is the optimal color. So if you find that drinking half your body weight in ounces of water per day causes your urine to be completely clear, you might consider drinking a little less.

## Workout hydration

Let's be honest: When most people go out for a run or a bike ride, they show little, if any, consideration for hydration. The only time people really pay any attention to hydrating during exercise is when they are doing a really long workout such as a 20-mile (32.2 km) run or 100-mile (161 km) bike ride (or at the gym, where you really don't need to carry water physically on your person). Other than that, there is usually little thought to hydration during workouts.

It's true that when your workout is shorter, your hydration needs are not as high, but they should still be taken into consideration based on the amount worked out. So during a one-hour workout, still hydrating 5 to 10 ounces (148 to 295.7 ml) every fifteen to twenty minutes may be important for you if it's particularly intense, you are a heavy sweater, and/or you are working out frequently. But realize that hydration is always important. If you engage in numerous workouts per week without properly hydrating, then you are constantly depleting your body of necessary fluids and electrolytes. Each successive workout only serves to deplete and dehydrate you even more. The problem is that most people don't recognize the symptoms of dehydration and often blame other things as a result. Fatigue, headaches, and runs that "feel harder than usual" are quite often a result of some level of dehydration.

We need to formulate our own personal hydration plan and put it into practice during our training. Just like our nutrition, finding what works for us when it comes to hydration takes time. We need to experiment with different amounts of fluid, different intervals for taking it in, and the kinds of fluids we consume, which may require different decisions for running, biking, and swimming.

## Thirsty? The controversy continues

One of the most hotly debated topics, even today, is whether or not you should drink before you are thirsty when it comes to exercise. It has long been said that if you wait until you are thirsty to drink, it is too late. You are already dehydrated.

There are those who take the opposite opinion, however, including some prominent sports scientists. They argue that our thirst mechanism is not flawed, that our bodies will tell us when it is time to drink, and there is no reason to do so beforehand. Listen to your body, they say. It knows all.

My take on it is to drink early and drink often. Don't wait until you are thirsty. Personally, I don't get thirsty that often at all. It usually happens for me after really long workouts in hot weather. If I truly waited to hydrate until I was thirsty, I would be in big trouble.

So I believe we need to hydrate with a set schedule, one that has been practiced and dialed in over time. It's better to be a little bloated rather than dehydrated and trying to catch up, especially during a race.

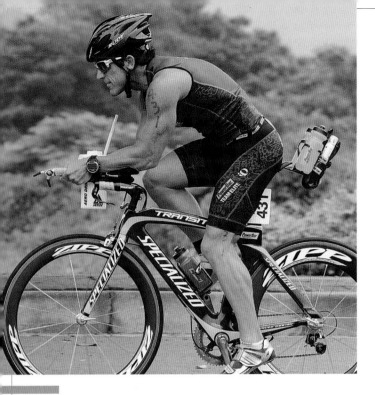

The author at Ironman
South Korea on Jeju Island.

## Long workouts

If you are training for the longer distance triathlons such as the half Ironman and Ironman distance races, you will most likely need to hydrate with more fluid than you can carry on the bike and the run. How do you get all the necessary fluids in? Here are two possible options:

1. **Stash fluids along your training course:** Especially useful for longer runs, you go out the night before and drop your fluid (and nutrition, if need be) at predetermined stops along your route. For example, if you are doing a 20-mile (32.2 km) run in preparation for an Ironman, you can stash fluids and gel every 5 miles (8 km) so you don't have to carry as much with you and can refuel at set intervals.

2. **Design your course with "aid stations" along the way:** This technique is great for fueling your multiple-hour bike training rides. When plotting your bike route, design it so that there is a gas station, convenience store, or water fountain at periodic intervals throughout your ride. Many Ironman races have aid stations every 20 miles (32.2 km) or so; if you are doing a 100-mile (161 km) training ride, you can make it so your refueling stop is every 20 miles (32.2 km) as well. Remember that the closer your training workouts are to your race-day plan, the greater success you will have.

## Hyponatremia

It's true, drinking too much water can be a bad thing, potentially life-threatening. Known as hyponatremia, or "water intoxication," this condition is characterized by dangerously low blood sodium levels. Cases of hyponatremia begin to increase as the number of people participating in events such as the marathon increased in popularity over the past decade. Triathletes and runners had obviously gotten the message about hydration, but then took it a little too far. People who experience hyponatremia generally share the following characteristics: They tend to overhydrate before the event, continue to hydrate excessively during the event itself, and were often out on the course for long periods of time without losing significant amounts of fluid through sweat. All of this excess water intake without a concurrent loss of water through sweating throws off the sodium balance in the bloodstream. You need not obsess about experiencing hyponatremia; the cases of it are somewhat rare. You just need to be sure not to overdo your water intake before and during the event. You should also try to use a sports drink containing sodium instead of exclusively drinking water to also protect the sodium balance in your body.

## MYTH: TAKING IN CAFFEINE DURING EXERCISE WILL CAUSE DEHYDRATION

**False.** It was commonly held that taking in caffeine during exercise would cause dehydration due to the caffeine's diuretic effect. Current research indicates that this is not the case. As I will discuss in the chapter on supplements, many endurance athletes utilize caffeine as an ergogenic aid, stimulating the central nervous system and helping our bodies to utilize fat as a fuel substrate. Soda with caffeine can be found at the run aid stations of most Ironman marathons, and many consume caffeinated beverages to help them through later stages of the marathon.

## Calculating your sweat rate

One very simple test to see how much water you lose during exercise is to weigh yourself before and after an exercise session. Weigh yourself naked before a workout of an hour in length; then weigh yourself naked again immediately afterward. You will most likely be amazed how you will have lost 1, 2, 3 pounds (0.5, 1, 1.4 kg) or even more.

If you *gain* weight during the workout, this means that you have consumed too much fluid.

The rule of replacing fluid post-workout is also simple. For every pound you lose, you want to replace it with a pint (16 ounces [473.2 ml]) of fluid. So if you lose 2 pounds (1 kg) during your workout, rehydrate with 2 pints (946.4 ml) of fluid afterward.

## Water or sports drink

Another common question is when to drink water and when to drink a sports drink during exercise. The general rule of thumb is that for workouts lasting less than an hour in normal conditions, water should be consumed. For workouts exceeding an hour, workouts in hot and humid conditions, or if you're a salty sweater, taking in a sports drink is recommended.

You may or may not be familiar with the term salty sweater. People who are salty sweaters generally know who they are. I myself am definitely one of them. You are a salty sweater if you have white stains on your dark-colored workout clothes and even your face and body after a particularly hot workout. These are salt stains, large amounts of sodium lost through sweat, and this indicates that you most likely need to supplement with sodium during these types of workouts.

Let's look at the specific elements found in the traditional sports drink:

1. Fluid
2. Electrolytes
3. Carbohydrates

Sports drinks provide us with three things that are essential to us as triathletes: fluid replacement, electrolyte replacement (especially sodium), and energy in the form of carbohydrates. Water only provides us with fluid.

## MYTH: THE SUGARS IN SPORTS DRINKS ARE BAD FOR YOU

**True** and **False:** If you're sitting on the couch and drinking a sports drink, then you have no need for the sugar. Have some water instead. If you were engaged in exercise requiring energy, however, especially extended exercise, then yes, this sugar is indicated. The sugar found in these sports drinks is just that, energy to fuel our exercise. They are not designed for and were never meant to be a leisurely beverage. They contain specific rapidly absorbed carbohydrates meant to provide a quick source of energy for our working muscles.

Remember that during workouts more than an hour, especially those lasting two, three, and four hours long, your body needs carbohydrates to replace the energy being burned off during exercise. After the initial hour of training, the general recommendation is thirty to sixty grams of carbohydrate an hour. Sports drinks are a great way to help provide the body with carbohydrates in addition to other sports foods such as GUs, energy chews, and sports beans.

An ideal sports drink has about fourteen to seventeen grams of carbohydrate in 8 ounces (236.6 ml), and anything much higher than that could possibly cause gastrointestinal distress. Some people can tolerate higher amounts, many cannot. For example, some athletes find they can't even tolerate the seventeen grams of carbs in Powerade, so they stop drinking a sports drink altogether, when if they would just drink a sports drink with fewer carbohydrates such as Gatorade, they might find they are okay.

So even though we think of hydration as primarily fluid replacement, it can and should be much more than that. The liquids we choose to hydrate with can also provide us with valuable energy and essential electrolytes. I am a big believer that, given the choice between water and a sports drink, the wiser choice is often the latter because it delivers so much more to our bodies than just fluid.

## Bathroom breaks on the bike

This chapter seems as good a place as any to tackle the oft-thought about but rarely broached subject, "How do I pee while on the bike?" Yes, especially for the longer-distance triathlons, nature will most likely call at least once if not several times during the bike leg.

First, let me begin by saying that this is not a bad thing or one to be avoided. I have heard triathletes say that they "hydrated perfectly" because they did not have to pee once during their race. Not having to urinate is not an indication that you hydrated perfectly—in fact, it can often mean the opposite.

### THE HISTORY OF GATORADE

In 1965, an assistant football coach at the University of Florida assembled a team of university physicians in an attempt to determine why the Gators players' performances suffered in the hot Florida conditions. The four researchers identified fluid and electrolyte losses as the two main causes along with carbohydrate depletion. They formulated a solution containing electrolytes and carbohydrates in the laboratory and named it Gatorade. The team's record began improving and, after the 1966 season, the Gators won the Orange Bowl for the first time in the school's history.

So what to do when nature calls while pedaling? You have two options:

1. **Use an aid station:** Most races will have Porta Potties (Porta Loos in the U.K.) at designated intervals along the course. Take the few seconds it takes to relieve yourself and use the first one you come across. Do not "hold it in" because this will only serve to stress your body more for the remainder of the race.

2. **Just go:** There, I said it. Yes, there are triathletes (myself included) who just pee while on the bike. If you are trying to turn in your fastest race time possible then stopping to go is generally not an option. Yes, like everything else in triathlon, this "technique" takes practice but it can be done. It can also be an effective technique to "discourage" those from illegally drafting behind you, so I killed two birds with one stone during one of my Ironman Florida races.

## Workout hydration guidelines

- 16 to 20 ounces (473.2 to 591.5 ml) of fluid one to two hours pre-workout
- 8 to 10 ounces (236.6 to 295.7 ml) of fluid ten to thirty minutes pre-workout
- 8 to 10 ounces (236.6 to 295.7 ml) of fluid every ten to twenty minutes during exercise
- 16 to 24 (473.2 to 709.8 ml) ounces of fluid for every pound (0.5 kg) lost during exercise
- 24 ounces (709.8 ml) of fluid for every pound lost during exercise if you are doing another workout that day

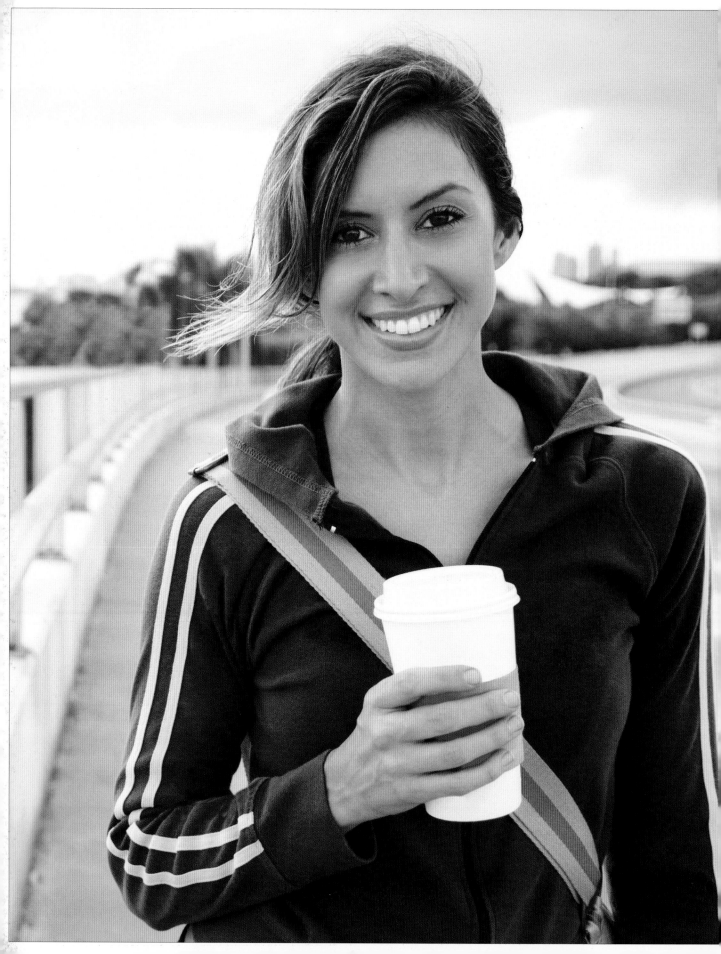

# Supplements and Ergogenic Aids

# CHAPTER 6

**ONE OF MY FIVE BROTHERS DECIDED HE** was going to "get ripped" a few years ago. He marched down to his local supplement store and dropped hundreds of dollars on a plethora of protein powders, pills, and the like. While he was religious about taking all of these new supplements with their flashy labels, he didn't really change his diet or his workouts, and he didn't really change his body as a result.

This was surprising to him. He expected a quick and significant return from his investment in these products, most of which promised huge results. He is far from alone. Millions of people are just like him, buying into the slick marketing hype of sports supplement companies, promising dramatic results.

Realize that there is no magic pill, powder, or potion when it comes to health, wellness, or sports performance. Not one. This goes for weight loss, muscle-building, and becoming a better athlete. Nothing takes the place of hard training.

You have to do the work.

Let me qualify that: There is no legal product that will provide significant benefit simply from taking it. Yes, there are now countless illegal substances that will make you a significantly better athlete simply by swallowing or injecting them. They are easier than ever to acquire thanks to the Internet and less-than-ethical doctors, and yes, their use is not just limited to the professionals any more. It may surprise you to know that even age-group triathletes (nonprofessionals) are now taking banned substances to improve their performance.

So what's the point in taking supplements? If there is no huge payoff, why waste the money? Especially when the efficacy of many of these supplements is still open to debate?

These are all great questions. There are some, doctors included, who believe that all you really get from taking supplements is "expensive urine." In other words, you pee out most of what you take in.

Love your java? Good news—
It helps sports performance.

I am the first to agree that many of the products on the market today are questionable at best. Walk into any supplement store and you are immediately overwhelmed by the sheer quantity of products of all shapes and sizes lining the shelves from floor to ceiling. I always feel bad for the person working behind the desk at these stores; there is absolutely no way he or she can possibly keep up with what even half of these products are claiming to do. He or she would need several Ph.D.'s in nutrition, chemistry, and exercise physiology to even begin to understand what all of the products' benefits and side effects might be.

So why take supplements at all if none of them acts as a "magic bullet" for the triathlete? Why waste time and money on something that won't catapult you to the next level? While there may not be one supplement that dramatically improves performance as a triathlete, there are a handful of products that, especially when

taken together, can in fact significantly improve your performance. Just like so many other things in exercise and fitness, it is the small things done consistently that bring about significant results, not any one thing done exclusively or occasionally.

My most successful clients are the ones who have been the best at consistently implementing these seemingly smaller things when it comes to their training: stretching, strength training, visualization, healthy eating, and, yes, supplementation. While supplements alone won't turn you into an uber triathlete, consistent, intelligent supplementation can indeed make a big difference in the quality of your workouts, the time to recovery, and your race results as well.

So what exactly is a supplement? When it comes to sports, a supplement is simply something used to enhance performance. They can include a wide variety of substances, including vitamins, minerals, herbs, commercially made powders, drinks, bars, pills, and the like.

A quick little history lesson: In 1994, the Dietary Supplement Health and Education Act (DSHEA) was passed, giving the Food and Drug Administration the job of regulating the supplement industry. The FDA regulates supplements using a different set of regulations than they do for foods and drug products, specifically that the manufacturer of a dietary supplement or ingredient is responsible for ensuring it's safe before it is marketed. The FDA therefore only takes action against any unsafe supplement after it is on the store shelves and is found to be unsafe.

## ERGOGENIC AID

What is an ergogenic aid? When it comes to sports, it is broadly defined as a substance or even a technique used to improve performance. It can be classified as nutritional, pharmacologic, physiologic, or psychologic.

That's a little frightening when you think about it. Pretty much anyone can come up with a new supplement, slap a label on it, and start selling it without any quality controls or testing whatsoever. Just a note of caution if and when you decide to purchase any supplements: It's a good idea to do your homework and research the specific product beforehand and to only use well-known brands and supplements that have been on the market for a long time.

Recent data reports that Americans spend roughly 11 billion dollars on supplements annually, with one in three people taking at least one nutritional supplement daily. What is pretty incredible is that sports supplementation is probably one of the least understood areas of sport nutrition.

When it comes to supplementation as triathletes, a distinction needs to be made between the supplements we take during our daily lives and the products we consume during our races. The products we take during our daily lives are generally for our overall health and well-being, while the other supplements are meant to help fuel our bodies during races.

As I have said before, I believe we should strive to get our nutrients from real food whenever possible. Food in its natural state is simply infinitely better than its synthetic counterparts. Unfortunately, it's not always possible to take in real food, whether it is due to travel, a busy schedule, dietary restrictions, etc. But I am a realist when it comes to what we can and cannot do, and if it means taking a commercially made supplement instead of nothing at all, then I believe in opting for the former.

Following is a list of the ten supplements I believe to be the most beneficial to the triathlete. It includes six supplements to take during daily living and training and four to consume during the race itself.

There are obviously dozens if not hundreds of other supplements I could have included on this list. But these are the ones with the most research behind them at this time and the ones that I believe to be the most efficacious to you as a triathlete and should therefore be the bedrock of your supplementation program.

## Supplements for daily life and training

### 1. PROTEIN POWDERS

One of the most popular and most effective supplements for both athletes and non-athletes alike is a commercially made protein powder. They come in a dizzying number of forms to choose from, including whey, soy, hemp, and pea, to name but a few. While research suggests that people generally get in the required amount of protein each day, I disagree with this statistic and believe it's most likely due to inaccurate self-reporting. As I discussed in the chapter on protein, endurance athletes' protein requirements are thought to be higher than the average person. We break down our muscles when we exercise, and dietary protein helps to rebuild and repair these muscles. Whey protein is the highest in branched chain amino acids (see chapter 3) and ideal for post-workout for those without a milk protein allergy.

Trying to reach our daily protein requirements from real food alone can be difficult, and whipping up a quick protein shake in a blender or even a shake bottle is an easy solution. Whether it's drinking a healthy protein shake with frozen fruit and omega-3 oil in the morning for breakfast or bringing a premade protein shake with you in your car so you can take it after your track workout, protein powders can be a simple, convenient, and relatively inexpensive way to ensure you are giving your body the protein it needs.

**Recommended Daily Intake:** 0.5 to 0.8 grams per pound (0.5 kg) of body weight

## 2. RECOVERY PRODUCTS

Triathletes by definition tend to work out frequently, often two times a day or more, depending upon your race distance and your goals. When sports scientists discovered the "metabolic window" not too long ago—the period of time after a workout that the body is best able to take in carbohydrates and protein—yet a new line of sport supplements was born. Recovery nutrition products' two main ingredients are carbohydrates and protein, anywhere from a 4:1 ratio to 7:1 ratio—carbs to restock the body's depleted energy stores in the form of glycogen and protein to help repair and rebuild muscle broken down by exercise. They may also have numerous other ingredients, including electrolytes, but the two things you are mainly looking for in a recovery product are carbohydrates and protein in the above-mentioned ratios. Ideally, you do not want much fat in a recovery product because fat slows down digestion; the post-workout goal is quick digestion, leading to quick absorption and thus recovery.

Recovery nutrition products come in all forms: premade recovery drinks, powders, bars, and so on. They are a very convenient and easy way to ensure that you not only get the most out of your workouts, but that you are also best prepared for your next workout as well.

**Recommended Daily Intake:** Post-workout caloric intake will vary based on numerous factors including body weight and duration and intensity of workout.

## 3. MULTIVITAMIN

I have to be honest: It drives me crazy when I hear people in the health and wellness community discourage the taking of a multivitamin because "you get all the vitamins you need in your healthy diet." I don't know too many people who eat that perfectly and, given the incredible number who are overweight, primarily from consuming large quantities of processed foods devoid of nutritional value, taking a multivitamin daily seems to be such a simple solution without any negative side effects. One small pill can help fill in the gaps in our nutrition, providing insurance when we fail to take in the necessary healthy nutrients.

Once again, nothing can compare to real food when it comes to the health benefits they confer. Science simply cannot harness all the incredible things that nature has to offer and condense them down into a pill form. Getting your vitamin C from a tablet is simply not the same as getting it from eating an orange. You should therefore strive to eat as much healthy food as often as possible, using a multivitamin only to help when your diet is lacking.

## 4. OMEGA-3 FATS

As I discussed in the chapter on fats, just like carbs, dietary fats have gotten a bad rap over the past few decades. And just like carbs, there are good fats and bad fats. Let me reinforce yet again how consuming foods rich in omega-3 fats such as salmon, tuna, walnuts, flaxseeds, chia seeds, and omega-3 fortified eggs have been shown to have a myriad of incredible health benefits, including the following:

1. Reduced inflammation of the arteries
2. Lowered blood pressure
3. Lowered triglyceride levels
4. Reduced risk of arrhythmia and sudden death
5. Reduced risk of blood clots

These are all amazing side effects of a healthy diet that includes omega-3 fats, especially the heart protective function. Research has indicated other potential benefits that are extremely beneficial to the endurance athlete and triathlete, including potentially:

1. Decreasing muscle soreness by decreasing inflammation
2. Reducing joint pain and stiffness

The potential benefits of a diet rich in omega-3 fats are enormous for both the average person and the endurance athlete alike. Since the side effects of omega-3 supplementation are essentially nil, you should strive to make these healthy fats a big part of your overall eating plan. Again, it is always best to try to get your nutrients from real food whenever possible, and this holds true for healthy fats as well. This is not always possible, however, so taking omega-3 supplements is an easy way to ensure you reap the powerful benefits of this nutrient:

**Recommended Daily Intake:** two to four grams

### OMEGA-3 FAT SUPPLEMENTS

1. **Flaxseed oil**
2. **Fish oil**
3. **Chia seeds**

### CHIA SEEDS

Chia seeds are a simple way to get in your omega-3s. Chia is an edible seed that comes from the desert plant *Salvia hispanica*. It is even more rich in omega-3 fatty acids than flaxseed. It is rich in antioxidants and fiber, along with a host of other beneficial nutrients. I often mix a few teaspoons (13 to 17 g) of chia into my oatmeal in the morning for a powerful start to my day. You can also mix either flaxseed or fish oil into protein shakes as well.

## 5. GLUCOSAMINE/CHONDROITIN

Almost 30 million adults in the United States suffer from osteoarthritis, a degenerative joint disease caused by the breakdown of cartilage within the joint. This cartilage serves to protect the bones from rubbing against one another, and when it begins to wear away, pain and loss of motion is often the result.

Glucosamine and chondroitin sulfate are natural substances found in and around the cells of cartilage. Glucosamine, an amino sugar, is a natural compound produced by the body and is found in cartilage. Chondroitin sulfate is a complex carbohydrate that helps the cartilage retain water.

While the studies are indeed mixed as they quite often are when it comes to the efficacy of a supplement, there is current research that indicates taking a combination of glucosamine sulfate and chondroitin sulfate may help alleviate joint pain and stiffness. It is also believed that they may not only help prevent the breakdown of joint cartilage, but may even help strengthen and rebuild it as well.

There are many within the medical community who do not believe in the benefits of glucosamine and chondroitin supplementation; there are also many who do. Those who do not believe in its effectiveness use the "expensive urine" description.

My take on it is this: If the research indicates that the side effects are minimal to none, and taking glucosamine and chondroitin might provide valuable insurance against age-related loss of cartilage, then why not? I'm willing to make that long-term investment.

I personally have never experienced joint pain due to osteoarthritis, so I take glucosamine and chondroitin proactively. Many who currently have pain and take the supplement insist that it does help with their symptoms. The results are not instantaneous, however, often taking weeks or even months to take effect.

So, as with any supplement, the choice is yours when it comes to taking glucosamine and chondroitin. Just know that it may help if you are currently experiencing osteoarthritic-type joint pain, and it may also help prevent the future breakdown of cartilage.

**Recommended Daily Intake:** 1,500 milligrams of glucosamine and 1,200 of chondroitin

## 6. BCAAS: BRANCHED CHAIN AMINO ACIDS

Branched chain amino acids have been one of the main supplements taken by strength athletes for their supposed ability to help minimize muscle damage as well as speed the recovery process. BCAAs include leucine, isoleucine, and valine, and they are now being used by endurance athletes for the same reasons, to potentially help protect muscle tissue, but from the damage caused by long-duration workouts rather than intense weight lifting sessions. BCAAs are reported to be significantly depleted during long bouts of exercise, and supplementation with them may have beneficial effects on the muscular system.

BCAAs may also positively impact the brain as well, with some studies suggesting that supplementation may improve mental function when fatigued, an important factor during longer distance triathlons when focus and mental toughness is needed.

BCAAs come either in pill or powder form. I find it easiest to take it in powder form by mixing it into my protein shakes.

**Recommended Daily Intake:** Five grams several times a day, ideally post-workout and right before bedtime.

In addition to supplementing your daily diet to maximize your training and overall health, you will also use a variety of sports supplements to fuel your triathlon on race day. Following are the four top supplements I recommend to get you to the finish line as fast as possible.

## 7. CARBOHYDRATE SOURCES

If you had to pick one dietary supplement as having the single greatest impact on triathlon performance, it would have to be carbohydrate products. Hands down. Carbs are our body's preferred source of energy, so it stands to reason that you better be sure to fill up your fuel tank with them.

By carbohydrate sources, I am referring to any food or fluids whose main ingredient is carbohydrate and is either consumed:

- **Pre-race:** To carbo-load, making sure fuel stores are full before the race starts
- **During the race:** To deliver fuel to the working muscles during longer distance triathlons

These carbohydrate products now come in an enormous variety of forms and flavors.

They can be powders, premade drinks, gels, sports beans, blocks, and bars. You need to determine what works best for you and stick with it. I will often refer to the three types of forms that these products come in throughout this book:

1. **Solid:** Think energy bars
2. **Semisolid:** Gels, blocks, and the like
3. **Liquid:** Sports drinks and other types of carbohydrate drinks

## 8. SPORTS DRINKS

In the previous chapter on hydration, I discussed the origin, uses, and benefits of consuming sports drinks during exercise. What amazes me is that there is still debate today on whether or not they help performance. Sports drinks provide our bodies with:

1. Fluid
2. Energy in the form of carbohydrates
3. Electrolytes

Sports drinks were not developed for the weekend warrior out for a leisurely round of golf. I don't care whether or not he's

### GUs

People often use the term "Goo" to refer to all energy gels: It is actually the name of one specific brand of energy gel, "GU."

carrying his bag instead of taking a cart, either. That's not exercise, and he doesn't need to hydrate with a sports drink. Water should do him just fine.

Somewhere along the line, the real use of sports drink became hijacked by the sports marketing industry. Suddenly everyone needed it to fuel their "sport," regardless of the type, intensity, or duration of the activity.

As I stated in the previous chapter, the sugars in sports drinks are not bad for you; they have a specific purpose—energy. These drinks are heavily tested in the laboratory, constantly refined, and made in such a way as to maximize intense, prolonged exercise. The types and combinations of sugars and the amount are specifically designed to empty from the stomach and be absorbed by the working muscles as quickly as possible, with the least amount of gastrointestinal distress.

Do you need to drink a sports drink during a 3-mile (4.8 km) power walk or hour-long indoor doubles tennis match? Probably not.

When it comes to exercise lasting over an hour, especially in hot and/or humid climates, sports drinks are a powerful supplement, helping to maximize performance. While originally created for football players, I would argue that they are even more beneficial to the triathlete exercising and racing in excess of an hour, often for five to fifteen hours or more.

We burn calories and we sweat out fluid and valuable electrolytes, three crucial things that these sports drinks provide. The longer and the more challenging the

conditions, the more important these three elements are to our overall success. You simply cannot continue to exercise when any one of these three things is severely depleted, much less all three.

Let's look at it another way: Is there any real downside from consuming a sports drink instead of water, especially during a long race? Why wouldn't you want the "insurance" of adding energy and electrolytes to your fluid, potentially avoiding having to slow down due to low fuel stores or painful muscle cramps?

To those who believe that water is just as effective if not more so than a sports drink when it comes to competing in endurance events such as triathlon, I like to say that I hope my competition only hydrates with water.

## 9. ELECTROLYTES

Many triathletes competing at the longer distances now take some type of electrolyte product during the race, with sodium being the primary ingredient. Electrolytes are lost in sweat, and the current wisdom held by triathletes and some exercise physiologists is that large losses of sodium can lead to debilitating muscle cramps on race day. Some sports scientists do not believe that sodium supplementation during an endurance event is warranted; many endurance athletes, professionals included, would strongly disagree with them.

Minerals in the blood and other body fluids that carry an electric charge (electrolytes) include sodium, potassium, and calcium. The level of electrolytes in the body is important for numerous bodily functions and processes, including muscular contractions. When our electrolyte balance is compromised, our performance can suffer.

Determining cause and effect when it comes to sports performance is extremely difficult, even when laboratory testing is involved. There are often too many variables to definitively compare what happens in experimental settings and state unequivocally that the same results will or will not occur under race conditions. Sports performance coaches must constantly compare and contrast the scientific evidence and anecdotal, looking for the best methods and techniques, which often fall somewhere in between the two.

In my research and personal experience, salt supplementation has proven to be one of the secrets to success at the longer-distance triathlons. I raced roughly ten Ironmans without taking in extra salt, and I experienced major muscle cramping. Once I began a strict salt supplementation strategy, I raced my next eleven with cramping not being an issue. Salt has been the single most effective supplement next to carbohydrates for me, as an athlete and as a coach.

Does this mean that low sodium is absolutely the sole cause of muscle cramping? No. It means that, for me and the hundreds I have coached to race long distances, salt supplementation has continually proven to be a positive part of our race supplementation strategy. It's not to say that the electrolyte potassium is not important; it is, but it is not the main culprit of cramping.

Potassium is another electrolyte that is essential to athletes. Though needed in smaller quantities than sodium, potassium is critical for fluid balance, especially during exercise. Think of sodium and potassium working in concert together to manage and regulate nerve impulses and muscle contraction. During exercise, more sodium is lost in sweat, which is why you might add salt to your water. If you look at a sports drink or product, you will find most have sodium and potassium, with sodium in greater quantities. Consuming potassium in these types of products should be sufficient, but you can also add potassium-rich foods to your diet such as strawberries, bananas, potatoes, spinach, avocado, milk, and yogurt. There is no need to add additional potassium to your workout drink.

Electrolyte supplements can include salt tablets, salt "sticks," and other similar type products. They are relatively difficult to find in supplement stores; many of the best brands must be purchased online as a result. One important note when it comes to salt supplements: Some of the more popular brands used by triathletes actually contain relatively little sodium chloride relative to other products. The one I use and recommend contains roughly 250 milligrams of sodium chloride, while the other popular brand contains less than half that, an amount that is too low in my experience given the dosage recommendations.

A general sodium recommendation is to take one gram per liter of fluid. You may need more or less, but this is a good starting point. I personally need more. Also, some triathletes with a family history of high blood pressure worry about their salt intake during exercise. This is generally not a concern; you still need the sodium because it is dependent upon the amount of salt sweated out during exercise.

## 10. CAFFEINE

Can caffeine help improve sports performance? Until 2004, it was banned in the Olympics at certain levels by WADA, the World Anti-Doping Agency. That should tell us something. These restrictions have since been lifted, and athletes in many sports continue to use caffeine to boost their performances. Even though it has been researched extensively, there is still some debate as to what if any benefits are derived from caffeine supplementation when it comes to sports.

Reportedly consumed by more than seventy-five percent of Americans on a daily basis and the most widely used drug in the world, caffeine is a mild stimulant that is found in nature in more than sixty plant species. It is also an ingredient in many commercial products including energy drinks, coffee, tea, and sports gels.

Used in moderation, recent studies show it may have significant health benefits beyond sports performance, including protection against certain age-related cognitive disorders.

When it comes to sports, the benefits of caffeine are mental as well as physical. The psychological benefits seem to come from the fact that it stimulates the central nervous system. This can translate into the following:

- Increased levels of concentration
- Decreased feeling of fatigue

Physiologically, caffeine may help increase performance by helping to mobilize fatty acids and increase their utilization as fuel. Remember that our bodies store significantly more fat than carbohydrate, but we simply cannot utilize this fat as a fuel as easily. Carbohydrates are our bodies preferred energy source, and when we run

### DIURETIC EFFECT DURING SPORTS

Some believe that the negatives outweigh the positives when it comes to caffeine supplementation for sports performance, focusing specifically on the diuretic effect associated with caffeine ingestion. While it is indeed true that one of the pharmacological actions of large doses of caffeine is increased urine output by the kidneys, the current research actually indicates that this is not an issue during sports performance, and caffeine supplementation does not decrease performance as a result of fluid losses. Again, I always go back to the professionals; if the vast majority of professional triathletes are using caffeine in some capacity, there must be performance-enhancing benefits.

out of them, we have problems. The ability to use fat a little bit more as a fuel source is a huge advantage to the endurance athlete because it will spare our carbohydrates so we have more energy to exercise longer.

Mentally stronger. Lessened feeling of fatigue. Better utilization of fat as a fuel. These are three incredible benefits to athletes in general and triathletes in particular, especially the long-distance triathlete.

As with everything you consume in your training and racing, you should experiment with caffeine if you decide to use it as part of your sports nutrition plan. People react to caffeine differently, and side effects can include gastrointestinal distress, something you definitely don't want to have happen during a race. In addition, on race day, you are likely to have more adrenaline circulating in your body, which also can make you feel more "jittery" and stimulate your central nervous system. Do not use caffeine on race day without having tested it out beforehand.

## Placebo effect

I cannot have a true discussion concerning sports supplements without bringing up the concept of the placebo effect. When it comes to sports supplementation, the placebo effect is defined as a beneficial result based not upon the specific properties of the product itself, but rather on the person's belief in the product.

There is nothing more powerful than the placebo effect when it comes to supplemen-

tation. In other words, a product may have an effect on you not because the active ingredients created a physiological response in your body, but rather because your belief that the product would work caused the positive effect. Scientists often give their subjects sugar pills and tell them that it is a certain type of medication that will have specific results, and the people often claim to experience these results even though they essentially took a "phony" pill.

The mind is so incredibly powerful and such a huge part of sports performance on many levels. I believe that harnessing the power of the body as well as the mind is the true secret to optimal sports performance. You cannot focus on just the body or the mind and reach your true potential. Every top athlete does some type of mental training as part of their preparation process, regardless of their sport.

The placebo effect is both a good and bad thing when it comes to sports performance. Why? Simple. Athletes will all too often ascribe positive effects to a product even though the product itself may have had absolutely nothing to do with that specific outcome.

But if they think it worked, then it did, right? So what's the problem?

The problem is that triathletes often try certain things during shorter workouts under more favorable conditions and experience positive effects, effects that most likely will not come during their longer race distances. So while the product may have worked once or twice because of the placebo effect, when

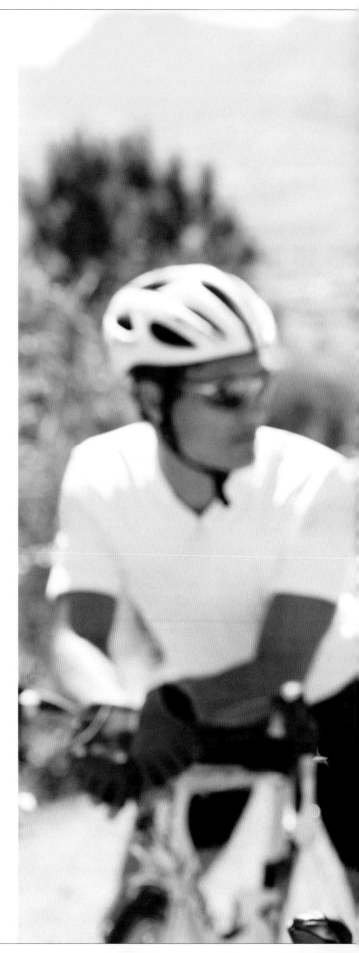

you really need it to work, say at mile 99 of the bike leg of an Ironman, the placebo effect might not be enough.

Throughout this book, I constantly talk about dialing in your race nutrition, the unending experimentation with various food, drinks, and supplements across numerous workouts so you can best determine exactly what works for you. One of the enormous challenges involved in this process is identifying the true cause and effect of all of these, determining what products, flavors, amounts, and timing intakes bring about your best performance, and what does not. A huge part of this constant experimentation is figuring out what effects come as part of the placebo effect and what is the result of the actual product itself.

As strong as the mind is, it can only take you so far.

Triathlon training involves constant experimentation and trial-and-error.

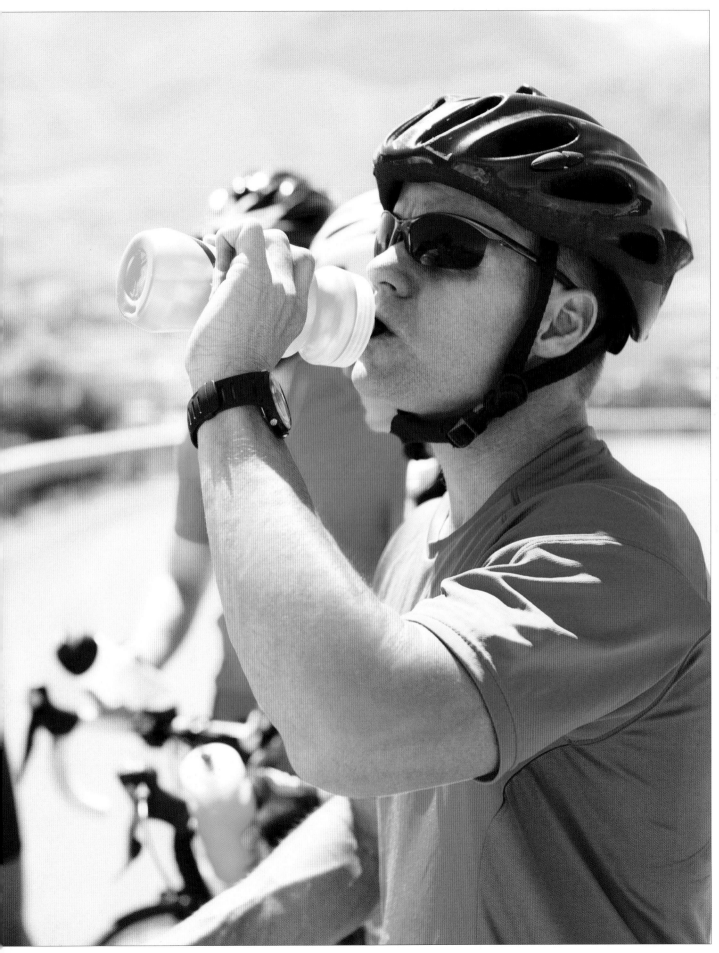

# PART 2

Training
_____

Fuel

# Dieting Down: Getting to Your Perfect Race Weight

**ONE OF MY FAVORITE THINGS ABOUT** triathlons is that they are truly the perfect fitness goal. Anyone who is familiar with goal setting knows that the best goals are challenging yet attainable and they have a specific date for achieving them. Triathlons fit these criteria perfectly for the vast majority of people, and they even grow with you. Your first goal may be to complete a sprint triathlon, and you may consider that to be a huge challenge at the time. Soon you have a few sprint triathlons under your belt, and before you know it, you're ready to jump up to the Olympic distance, then the half Ironman, and so on.

The vast majority of clients I've worked with over the years have named weight loss as one of their primary fitness goals. It's part of the human condition; we all think we could stand to lose weight, whether it be 100 pounds (45.4 kg), 50 (22.7 kg), or just 5 (2.3 kg). You, too, may be doing your triathlon as a springboard to lose weight. What better way to get in shape than being forced to swim, bike, run, and lift weights for an upcoming fitness event, right?

Even though you may start your triathlon training focused on your weight loss goal, the weight loss focus becomes less important as your training evolves, and before long, the goal of completing your triathlon takes precedence. You are no longer so invested in losing weight just to make the scale move. Rather, you train to complete an event to the best of your abilities, knowing that the more weight you lose, the faster you will go and the better experience you will have. That's pretty great.

Triathletes generally fall into two categories: participants and performers. They include those who want to cross the finish line and those who want to go as fast as they possibly can. Regardless of the goal, both groups will generally lose weight during their training. Your body doesn't care what your end goal is; cross-training for three different sports will torch some serious calories. Yet the simple physics remain: The lighter you are, the faster you will go.

Let me say again that many people are under the misconception that people who exercise frequently can eat whatever they want. This couldn't be further from the truth. The math just doesn't add up. The average person will burn roughly 600 calories per hour during running. All it takes is one Grande Frappuccino from Starbucks, and you've completely negated the effects of this workout. Face it, it is easy to "out-eat" your workout. So even though burning calories through exercise is an important component of weight loss for triathletes, it is just a piece of the puzzle—a much smaller piece than most people think. Most fitness professionals would agree that losing weight is somewhere around 80 percent nutrition and 20 percent exercise.

Don't misunderstand me: Burning calories through exercise is an important part of losing weight during your training. But to truly make the scale move and drop significant weight by race day, you have to focus on your day-to-day nutrition. No amount of working out will offset a bad diet. Unless of course you're Michael Phelps. But you're not, so it's a moot point.

## Evaluating your race weight

Way back in 2001, I was training for my third Ironman to be held on the island of Langkawi in Malaysia. I just completed Ironman Florida in around 10½ hours, and I really wanted to break 10 hours at this next Ironman. Understanding that the lighter I was, the faster I would go, I picked an extremely low body weight number and set out to achieve that weight by race day.

I severely restricted my calories while drastically increasing my training volume and intensity. When race day arrived, I had in fact achieved my arbitrarily chosen race day weight.

My swim was actually my fastest to date, so I was pretty excited as I mounted my bike to begin the 112-mile (180.3 km) bike ride. My excitement was short lived, however. Just a few miles down the tropical tree-lined highway, I was finished. My legs felt like they were made of iron and would barely move. Just to turn the pedals a few revolutions was a major undertaking. I was experiencing a bonk of epic proportions, before the race had even really started. I had absolutely no gas in my fuel tank and well over 100 miles (161 km) left to go.

I did end up finishing, but it was my toughest race by far. I learned a huge lesson that day about how picking an arbitrary weight loss number is a flawed approach. I may have hit my target weight, but I had completely overshot my body's preferred race weight. Remember that weight and performance are a J-shaped curve, meaning that some weight loss is good and will likely benefit or improve your performance. However, too much weight loss can actually negatively affect your performance. So when planning your race weight, it needs to be one that is achievable with adequate nutrition to fuel and refuel training on a daily basis.

Unfortunately, so many triathletes continue to make the same mistake I made that day: Take a seemingly random number that they would like to weigh for their triathlon and set out to achieve that goal, even though that weight may hamper rather than help their performance. Just like it's better to be 5 percent overtrained than 1 percent undertrained when it comes to racing, the same holds true with weight loss. In other words, it's exponentially better to be a few pounds over your ideal race weight than one pound underneath it. Overshooting your body's preferred race weight by just a little bit can have disastrous consequences.

Let's be realistic. If you know you're 40 pounds (18 kg) overweight, choosing a race day weight that is 20 pounds (9 kg) lighter is appropriate. If you're training 16 weeks for your triathlon, that means your goal is to lose a little over a pound per week, which is well within the healthy range and completely doable.

The problem with picking an arbitrary number applies mainly to the performers, those of you who are already fit yet want to lose those last few pounds. It is this group that is most at risk of overshooting their healthy race weight.

So if you know you have more than a few pounds to lose, and your goal of weight loss falls well within that range, it's okay to pick a race day weight loss goal. Just be sure it's well within that conservative range. What should this range be? You can start by using the "ideal body weight" equation for what a healthy weight is. For women, it is 100 pounds (45.4 kg) for the first 5 feet (1.5 m) and 5 pounds (2.3 kg) for every additional inch (25.4 mm). For men, it is 106 pounds (48 kg) plus 6 pounds (2.7 kg) for every additional inch (25.4 mm). Then for both, you have a range of +/- 10 percent in either direction. For example: For a 5-foot

(1.5 m), 6 inch (152.4 mm) woman, her ideal weight is 130 pounds (59 kg) with a healthy weight range of 13 pounds (6 kg) either direction, so a healthy weight range is 117 to 143 pounds (53 to 65 kg). This allows for body fat and bone structure differences. I believe that there is huge value in achieving that weight loss goal for your race, and it can give you a great deal of confidence during the race itself.

The great news is that, presuming you don't overdo it, every single pound you lose for your race will make you go faster. Just a few pounds lost can make a big difference in your finishing time. So if you lose some weight, even if it's not your intended amount, it's still a big accomplishment.

## Weight loss that works

In chapter 1, I began a discussion about the healthy way to lose weight. I have a bit of experience with this topic on a number of fronts: I have trained hundreds of people whose primary goal was weight loss; I have experimented with weight loss myself to get as light as possible for well over 100 marathons, ultramarathons, and Ironman triathlons, and as a Wilhelmina fitness model, I have had to "get ripped" for numerous DVD, television, and print photo shoots. I even did natural bodybuilding for a year back when I was a trainer in New York City (I hope those pictures never surface), where I really learned what obsessively clean eating is all about. All those experiences along with my master's studies in exercise science and my being certified as a sports nutritionist have allowed me to understand weight loss in a complete way.

Let me begin by stating that I don't believe in restrictive diets. I believe in healthy eating. "Dieting down" and "diets" are two completely different concepts. When dieting down with a fad diet, the only person who comes out ahead in the end is the author of the diet book you are following. Any eating plan that restricts entire food groups and has an end date is flawed from the very start. What works long-term is "eating clean" the majority of the time, eating healthy at least 80 percent of the time for health and performance and the other 20 percent for pleasure. This is "real-life" eating.

The weight loss that comes as a result of these crash diets is actually counterproductive, especially to the triathlete. First, much of the initial pounds dropped are water weight, not fat. Do the math: Let's say you lose eight pounds in one week, primarily through a fad diet alone.

### 8 pounds (3.6 kg) × 3,500 calories per pound = 28,000 calories lost

Do you really think you created a negative caloric balance of almost 30 thousand calories in one week? That comes out to a 4,000 calorie deficit per day. What you are seeing on that scale is lots of water loss, a little fat loss, and most likely a little muscle loss as well. Weight is made up of muscle, bone, water, and body fat, and technically you only want to lose one of those things. Weight on a scale is not the only variable; body fat testing is a much more accurate way of monitoring progress.

The muscle loss is a huge problem. The longer a person stays on one of these restrictive diets, the more muscle that is lost due to inadequate caloric intake. Our metabolisms are directly connected to the amount of lean muscle mass we possess. The more lean muscle mass we have, the higher our metabolisms are and the more calories we burn twenty-four hours a day. This is why it is so incredibly important that we preserve and preferably add to our muscle mass.

It's an insidious cycle. You go on a crash diet for a few weeks and lose a bunch of weight quickly. Part of the weight loss is from muscle, so now you have in effect lowered your metabolism. Your body will burn fewer calories throughout the day. So, when you inevitably stop dieting and go back to eating the exact same amount you were before, you begin to gain it all back. This is the horrible cycle of the crash dieter, constantly lowering their metabolisms through loss of muscle.

So how the heck do you lose weight then? The concept is actually really simple; it's the application that people have the most difficulty with. The secret is to eat better.

You set out to eat "cleaner," not necessarily less. I have yet to meet anyone who eats "perfectly," so we can all stand to improve upon our eating habits. When you start to cut back on the junk and focus on eating

It's simple physics. The lighter you are, the faster you go.

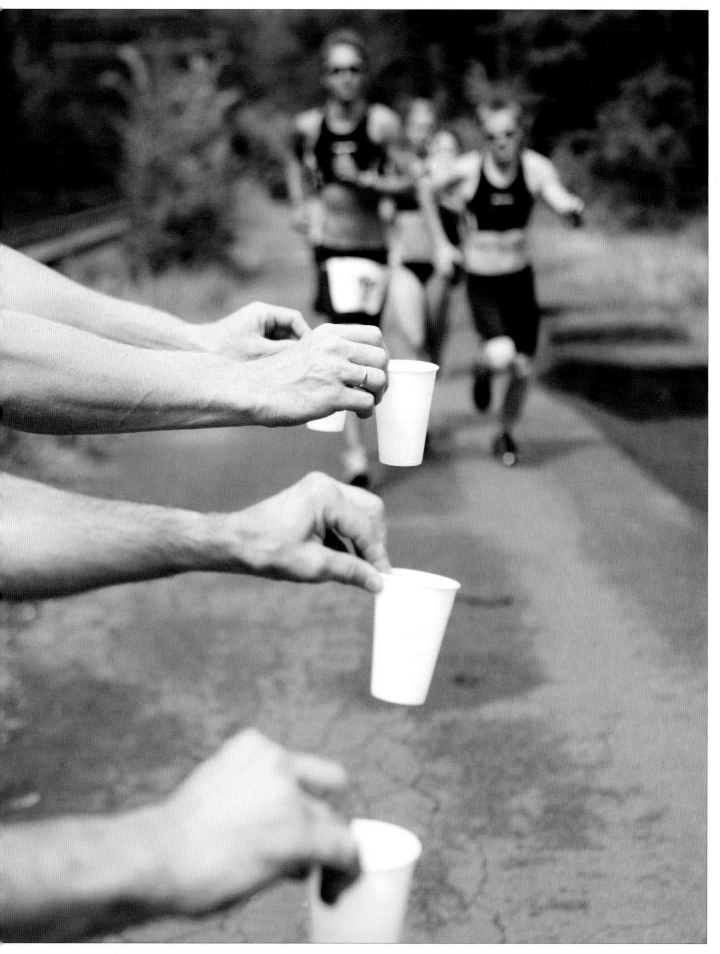

healthier, you will lose weight without focusing on caloric restriction. I discuss clean diets and better eating habits in chapter 8: Fueling Your Workouts.

## Weighing yourself

I recommend weighing yourself once per week. That's it. I know many of you probably want to get on that scale every single day, but I strongly recommend against it. Yes, there is even some research that shows weighing yourself every day has its potential advantages. I disagree.

Once again, it goes back to simple math, and the fact that 1 pound (0.5 kg) equals 3,500 calories. If you weigh yourself every day and see a loss (or gain) of a pound (0.5 kg) or more from one day to the next, it will be primarily from fluid loss rather than fat loss, unless you are significantly overweight. If true quality weight loss for the vast majority of people is 1 to 2 pounds (0.5 to 1 kg) per week, then if you climb on the scale every day, you will not see any major changes in a twenty-four hour period.

I recommend weighing yourself every Monday morning—first thing in the morning, right after you have gone to the bathroom. Your ultimate goal if you are trying to lose weight is to see the number on the scale drop by a pound or two (0.5 to 1 kg) each week. Remaining the same weight on a subsequent weigh-in is not the end of the world, either. If the scale doesn't move, then you simply need to tweak your eating toward being even healthier for the upcoming week.

The best scale shows weigh-in pounds as well as body-fat percentage. There are a wide variety of scales on the market today that provide these metrics and lots more. These are great tools to gauge your progress and keep you motivated.

Body fat is more important than pure weight loss over time. Ideally, you want both numbers to drop; you may, however, build some muscle during your training that will add some weight without adding to your body fat percentage.

## Muscle weight

A few years ago, I went into the laboratory at Adelphi University to get my VO2 max tested and my bike and run zones dialed in as well. After my tests were completed, I sat down with the exercise physiologist to discuss my results. His very first recommendation to me was to "lose the muscle." My years of strength training had added more than a few extra pounds of muscle, much more than your typical runner or

### VO2 MAX

VO2 max stands for maximal oxygen uptake and refers to the amount of oxygen your body is capable of utilizing. It is a measure of your capacity for aerobic work and can be a predictor of your potential as an endurance athlete.

triathlete. Even though my body fat percentage was low, my BMI actually put me in the overweight to obese range due to my muscle mass.

BMI is a great measurement of health and disease risk for the average person, but those who are leaner and have more muscle mass might be higher on a BMI chart. That does not necessarily mean that they are at a greater risk for disease, it just means that the dense muscle makes their weight on a scale higher. Again, this is why your weight alone is not always a true indicator of your overall body composition and why you should also always take into account your percentage of body fat.

I am a firm believer that strength training is an essential component of success in triathlon. Current research indicates that strength training improves performance, including improved running economy.

Strength training also benefits injury prevention. We all have weak links in our kinetic chain, and focused sport-specific strength training helps to eliminate these weak links, allowing us to train and race injury-free. I believe this is even more important than improvements in other areas such as running economy. If we can stay-injury free, we can continue to train.

But I knew the exercise physiologist was absolutely correct. I needed to get lighter if I wanted to get faster, and a big part of this for me would come from losing muscle weight. Did I stop strength training altogether? Absolutely not. I just changed what I was doing. When the time came to begin training for my next Ironman, I switched from a traditional bodybuilder's workout to a triathlon-specific strength workout. This workout was considerably shorter and much more functional, with the focus taken off of the upper body workout, or "vanity" type workout. The focus instead was on a lower body and core routine, with lighter weights and upper body exercises that were to improve swimming and running, not to build muscle.

So if you're someone who has been working out with the main goal of "muscle hypertrophy," namely building significant amounts of muscle mass, you may want to consider changing around your routine to a more triathlon-specific routine. You don't want to stop strength training by any means; you just want to change the reason why you are lifting weights. You can always go back to your former routine after your race is over.

## BMI CHART

Body Mass Index (BMI) is a number calculated from a person's weight and height. It is calculated by dividing weight in pounds by height in inches squared and multiplying by a conversion factor of 703.

| BMI | Weight Status |
| --- | --- |
| Below 18.5 | Underweight |
| 18.5 – 24.9 | Normal |
| 25.0 – 29.9 | Overweight |
| 30.0 and above | Obese |

Example: Weight = 185 pounds,
Height = 5 foot 8 inches (68 inches)
Calculation: $[185 \div (68)^2] \times 703 = 28.12$

## PROTEIN SHAKE

When I use the term protein shake, it does not mean protein only. I am referring to protein powders mixed with whatever liquids and extra ingredients you choose. Different brands have different amounts of protein and carbs in them, and when you add additional ingredients such as berries into the mix, you are adding more carbs as well. The ratio of protein to carbs depends upon your specific nutritional needs, goals, and the workout involved.

Here are 10 great carbohydrate and protein combo snacks:

1. Low-fat Greek yogurt and berries
2. 100 percent whole wheat crackers and a 2 percent string cheese
3. One slice 100 percent whole wheat bread and 1 tablespoon (16 g) peanut butter
4. Fifteen grapes and seven small cubes of 2 percent cheese
5. One medium apple and fifteen to twenty almonds
6. High-fiber granola bar and 8 ounces (236.6 ml) low-fat milk
7. Energy bar with protein and carbohydrates
8. Low-fat cottage cheese and ½ cup (75 g) chopped fruit
9. 6-inch (15.2 cm) whole wheat tortilla with 2 ounces (56.7 g) turkey/chicken and one slice 2 percent cheese
10. Turkey jerky and a fruit

## The basic eating plan

I recommend eating five to six medium-size meals throughout the day. A typical day might look like this:

**Meal #1:** 7:00 a.m. Breakfast
**Meal #2:** 10:00 a.m. Protein shake
**Meal #3:** 1:00 p.m. Lunch
**Meal #4:** 4:00 p.m. Fruit and peanut butter
**Meal #5:** 7:00 p.m. Dinner
**Meal #6:** 9:00 p.m. Protein shake

It looks like a lot of eating because it is scheduled eating. Most people "graze," eating throughout the day, taking in hundreds of calories, almost unconsciously. So often when I give this eating plan to someone who wants to lose weight, they say, "Oh, that's too much eating for me."

Really? Too much eating? If these people were in fact eating less, they wouldn't have to lose weight. Most people wait until they are hungry to feed themselves, and that's when we overeat as well as make poor food choices. The goal is to feed our bodies constantly with quality food sources containing slow-absorbing carbohydrates along with protein, avoiding sugar crashes and the subsequent feeding frenzy that soon follows. The more often you eat, the less hungry you will likely be, which should help with portion control throughout the day. Eating frequently also keeps blood sugar stable, which also stabilizes energy over the course of the day.

## The food journal

Personal trainers, nutritionists, coaches, and similar-type health professionals will often ask clients to keep a food journal for a few days so they can see what the client is eating, evaluate their diet, and make the necessary interventions.

It's ridiculous.

Some of the greatest works of fiction ever written have been food journals. Let's be real: People are not honest about what they eat—not even close. No one wants to admit how the wheels fell off the night before, and they ate a whole box of Mallomars. It's embarrassing.

If these food journals are remotely close to being factual, it's not because it's a true picture of the person's normal eating habits. It's because the person completely changed what they eat during the journaling period. So it's not a real snapshot of what the client eats on a day-to-day basis. It's the client altering their eating habits for a few days so as to not embarrass themselves.

Now, after all that, it might come as a shock when I say that you should consider keeping a food journal. Why? Because it's for you and you alone. You are not going to show it to anyone. When I went through my bizarre natural bodybuilding phase, I kept a food journal and was absolutely shocked at how much more I ate than I thought. We simply are unaware of how much food passes our lips on a daily basis: a handful of this; a sip of that; a bite or two of something else. BLTs—bites, licks, and tastes—add up to lots of calories over the day.

So the journal is for you to become aware of just how much more you are eating than you think you are—because you are, trust me. Try writing down everything you eat and drink for a full three days. EVERYTHING. This means every single solid or liquid that passes over your lips. You will be truly amazed at what you discover about your nutritional habits if you truly eat as you normally do.

## What to cut out

### PEANUT BUTTER

If I were stranded on a deserted island and was only allowed to eat one thing, it would be peanut butter. There's no question. I love it, I eat it almost daily, and when I do, my sandwiches are obscenely large. So when it comes time for me to start dieting down for an event, I cut out the peanut butter. It is a torturous process but necessary because I have identified the elimination of peanut butter sandwiches as one of the simplest ways for me to cut significant calories from my diet. By eliminating this one habit alone, I have immediately started to create a significant caloric deficit in my normal eating habits.

Realize that this specific change, eliminating peanut butter, worked for me and might not work for everyone. A teaspoon (5 g) of peanut butter can actually be helpful when people are trying to lose weight as a part of snack or a meal because the protein and fat help them feel more satisfied, and it does provide healthy fats, which lots of people miss over the course of the day.

So what is your personal "peanut butter?" Is there one thing you eat frequently that you can replace with a healthier or less calorically-dense alternative? Changing a "guilty pleasure" in your diet is one of the simple tricks to losing weight without dramatically altering your eating habits.

## ALCOHOL

One of the more common questions I receive about fitness and nutrition has to do with the consumption of alcohol. What's the best to drink if I'm trying to lose weight? Is beer better than wine? Is wine better than hard alcohol? Can I drink it at all?

As usual, moderation is key. Like caffeine, alcohol consumed in moderation has numerous health benefits. In fact, in 1992, Harvard researchers stated that moderate alcohol consumption was one of the "eight proven ways to reduce coronary heart disease risk." Other potential benefits include reducing the risk of a heart attack, stroke, and type 2 diabetes.

And now back to the math. Alcohol has seven calories per gram. That's three calories more than protein and carbs and two calories less than fat. Also, alcohol cannot be converted to glycogen and utilized as that source of fuel, so it must be stored as fat. That's not good when we're talking about maintaining your body's preferred weight.

So cutting back on or cutting out alcohol is one easy way to start to reduce your weekly caloric intake. If you drink two glasses of wine a night, consider cutting back to one.

## JUNK FOOD

There is no easier way to start on the path to healthy eating and weight loss than to keep the junk food out of the house. We still can have treats; we just need to get in the car and go to the ice cream store to enjoy them. As I tell my sons, if you have them every day, they are no longer "treats."

So if you are training and trying to also lose weight, focus on these ten tips to lose weight and improve your training:

1. Eat small meals frequently, including a carbohydrate (whole grain or fruit) and a protein (lean meat, low-fat dairy, egg, nuts, seeds, or beans).

2. Don't skip breakfast! Breakfast should be a base of whole grain carbohydrate, lean protein, and healthy fat. Don't just grab a granola bar or yogurt; you need a complete breakfast!

3. Be sure to include a post-workout shake or snack. Oftentimes, skipping this sets you up to be starving later.

4. Hydrate throughout the day with low-calorie beverages such as water, or a low-calorie sports drink if you need more electrolytes, and lightly flavored waters.

5. Don't drink your calories! Drinks such as soda, juices, some smoothies, fancy coffee beverages, sweet tea, etc., can add up to lots of extra calories that don't make you feel full.

6. Decrease or avoid alcohol intake when trying to lose weight or improve training. Alcohol causes dehydration and can add up to unwanted calories over the course of the day.

7. Avoid foods that are high in calories and low in nutrients such as fried foods, sugary processed foods, and baked goods.

8. If you are hungry after dinner or late at night, eat a small protein-rich food item such as a string cheese, low-fat Greek yogurt, or a handful of almonds, drink a glass of water, and wait fifteen minutes.

9. If you "mess up" on one meal, don't abandon the whole day! Make sure the rest of your meals and snacks are full of protein, fiber, and nutrients.

10. Follow the "80/20 Rule": 80 percent of the time focus on nutrient-rich foods that fuel your performance and 20 percent of the time include some pleasure foods. Remember, eat what you want, not everything you want!

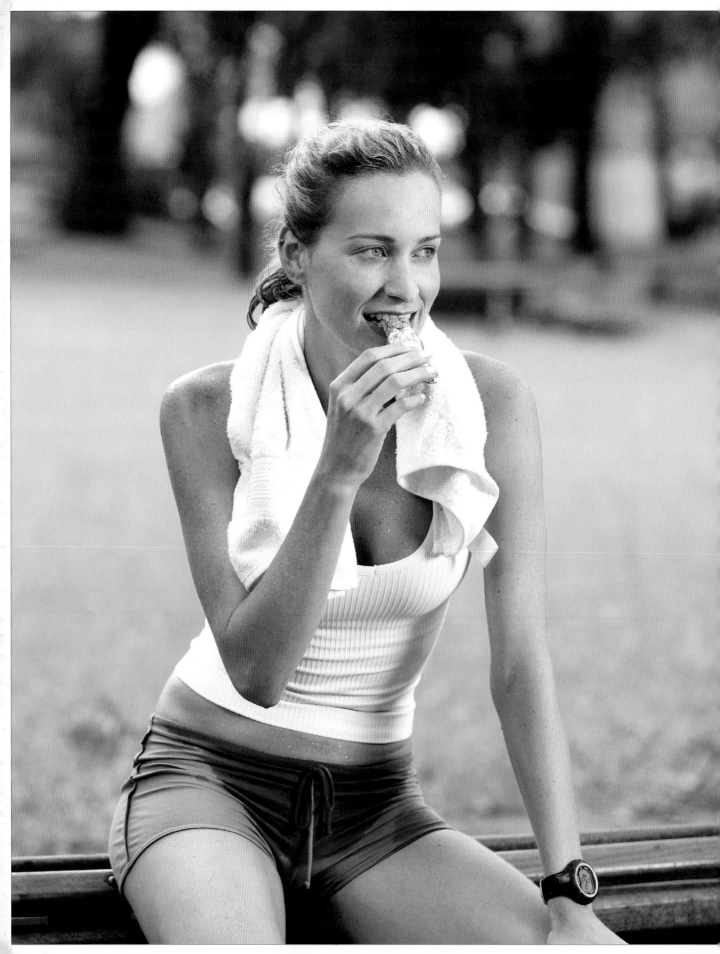

# Filling the Tank: Fueling Your Workouts

**IN CHAPTER 7, I TALKED ABOUT HOW** to get down to your perfect race weight—in essence, how to eat less and exercise more. In this chapter, I'll talk about fueling your workouts—how to eat more to exercise more. Yes, it would seem that the two concepts completely contradict each other. On the one hand, you want to eat less to get down to your ideal race weight, yet we still need to give our bodies the fuel they need to get through each and every workout session. If this seems a little complicated, it's because it is. Just look at the professional triathletes; they are constantly struggling to get down to their lightest possible weight while still consuming enough food to fuel their high-volume and high-intensity workout programs. This is difficult to do, especially at the professional level. Many pros end up dropping out of races because they have dieted down too hard and overshot their body's optimal race weight. They simply don't have the energy needed to deliver the power and speed required on race day.

Realize that there is no one-size-fits-all eating plan. What works for one person may be disastrous for another. There is a lot of variation in people's metabolic needs, and there are variations in the type of workouts that triathletes engage in. This complicates the issue exponentially. This is again why I recommend keeping a log of your training that includes your food intake as well. This food tracking will allow you to see patterns over time, giving you the valuable information you need to dial in your best possible personal nutrition strategy.

It may also seem confusing when I continually talk about eating five or six smaller meals spread out throughout the day. Does this schedule include fueling for the workouts and refueling after as well? The short answer is yes, it does. It just takes a little more planning around these workouts to optimally fuel up for them (and recover from them) while adhering to this multiple meal strategy. But it can be done.

Training for three different
sports requires fuel. Lots of it.

One of the most important things you will hear over and over again when it comes to nutrition is to listen to your body. You have to really get to know yourself inside and out if you want to perform at your best. This is because determining causality when it comes to sports nutrition is extremely difficult. It takes significant time, lots of patience, and a very open and unbiased mind. It is a constant experiment in an almost completely uncontrolled environment.

Take the example of someone training for an Ironman triathlon. They might use a new orange sports drink during their first long training run and experience stomach cramps during the workout session. When the run is over, they crash on the couch dejected and completely blame the orange sports drink for their gastrointestinal distress and sub-par run. They might blame just the orange flavor, or they might blame the specific brand of sports drink itself. I hear things like this all the time: "I can't use the Cherry AlligatorAid at all. I tried it once during a race, and it was horrible. It made me want to throw up."

Sure, maybe the specific sports drink is to blame for that person's cramping. But it's usually not that simple. Maybe what they ate before the run is truly to blame. Maybe they drank too much sports drink each time or maybe they drank too frequently. Perhaps it was an extremely hot day, and the heat itself was to blame for their discomfort. Maybe they just weren't used to running and drinking at the same time, which is quite often the case, especially for newer runners and triathletes.

The bottom line is that determining what works and what doesn't work when it comes to nutrition is very rarely a one-time experiment—or even a two- or three-time one at that. Determining causality takes significant trial and error with multiple "experiments" performed over time.

This same person may very well go out on a second long run utilizing the exact same product in the exact same way and have a fantastic workout. Does that mean that it does work for her? Maybe, maybe not. The smart thing for her to do in that case would be to look at what she ate prior to the first workout when she experienced gastrointestinal distress and see if that might have been the possible cause. Or maybe she ate the same thing before this workout as well, so perhaps she is just getting more acclimated to taking in fluids while running. The bottom line is that you simply cannot make quick determinations about what does and does not work for you nutritionally. There are far too many variables involved. This is why sports nutrition can be so incredibly tricky.

When we are talking about fueling your workouts and filling your tank, we are actually talking about two different time periods: what you fuel up with *before* your workouts and what you take in *during* the workout itself. As you get better at doing both of these things, you will feel better and you will perform better, a sign that you have started to dial in your sports nutrition plan.

## Workout fuel

There are three common questions asked when it comes to fueling our workouts:

1. What should I eat?
2. How much should I eat?
3. When should I eat?

Then there's also hydration questions as well. They are actually usually the exact same questions:

1. What should I drink?
2. How much should I drink?
3. When should I drink?

We learned in chapter 2 that our body's preferred energy source is carbohydrates, and that's part of the answer to question number one about eating. Carbs are the endurance athlete's best friend. We cannot live without them. We need them. They fuel our muscles and are therefore a huge part of our pre-workout fueling strategy.

## Exercising on an empty stomach

There still exists a debate within the fitness industry about whether or not it is best to work out on an empty stomach first thing in the morning, especially when fat loss is the goal. The argument is that, if you work out after fasting all night when your carbohydrate stores are depleted, your body must therefore utilize your fat stores as an energy source.

Sounds logical, right? Don't eat before your morning workout and burn fat instead of carbohydrates. Remember, though, that our bodies store literally thousands of

calories' worth of energy in the form of fat. Unfortunately, fat is not our body's preferred source of energy. We simply cannot burn it as a fuel as easily as we can carbohydrates.

Research appears to suggest that if we do work out on an empty stomach, our workouts may suffer. We may not be able to work out as long or at high intensities. We may not burn as many calories due to inadequate fueling. So it's not as simple as not eating before a workout in order to maximize fat and therefore weight loss. When total calories burned is the ultimate end goal, then eating before the workout seems to be warranted.

Here's where it starts to get tricky for us as triathletes: We ideally want to accomplish both competing interests at the same time, namely fueling our workouts while getting down to our optimal race weight. We don't want to over-fuel, but we don't want to under-fuel, either. We want to get the most out of our sessions without lessening the caloric expenditure and subsequent quality weight loss.

Here's the truth: I believe that workouts of one hour or less that are not extremely intense do not necessarily need fueling beforehand. You need to listen to your body over time and determine what it needs. If you are getting up at 6 a.m. to go out on an easy 6-mile (9.7 km) run, a pre-workout meal is not absolutely required. It all goes back to listening to your body. Swimming for thirty minutes? You may find you get stomach cramps if you eat anything too close to these workouts, so fueling up beforehand may not be for you.

If you engage in certain workouts without fueling up beforehand, and you noticeably suffer as a result, either during the workout itself and/or afterward, then you should consider fueling up for them beforehand. If you lack the energy to get through the workout, it may mean you need more fuel in the tank before you start. If you feel overly spent afterward, this may be a sign you need to fuel up beforehand as well.

Drinking a sports drink with carbohydrates might be helpful if you do not feel like eating before a workout because it will provide some carbohydrate for energy. In addition, you don't have to eat a whole meal before a 6-mile (9.6 km) run. If eating a meal does not sit well with your stomach, try a pre-workout snack of carbohydrate and a little protein. Here are five fueling pre-workout snacks:

1. Energy bar (ideally maybe 150 to 200 calories, twenty to forty grams carbohydrate, ten grams protein or less, and a few grams of fat)
2. One medium banana with a smear of peanut butter
3. Small baggie of dry whole grain cereal (three grams fiber or less per serving for pre-workout snack)
4. One slice wheat bread with a thin smear peanut butter
5. Granola bar with a few grams protein

I realize there are many people who find fueling up before workouts to be problematic. Doing so causes them discomfort, in the form of cramping, nausea, diarrhea, or some other type of gastrointestinal distress.

They tend to want to go into their workouts on an empty stomach without having eaten anything beforehand. What are these people to do? They need to listen to their bodies and determine what works for them and when. They have to adequately fuel themselves as well. Remember that over time, the body will likely adjust to what you give it. So just like you train the body to run or bike hard in the morning, it is also possible to train your body to have a snack or meal before that workout. Sometimes the key is starting small. For example, you eat half a bar each day for a week or two, then work up to eating three-quarters of the bar, and then finally the entire bar. Train the body to be able to handle pre-workout nutrition just like you train it to run faster and pedal harder.

## Becoming a fat-burning machine

Adequately fueling our workouts as triathletes is indeed essential, especially for our longer workouts. But wait. There is value to occasionally working out with a limited fuel supply. What does that mean? It means occasionally going out for a long run or bike ride and not fueling as much during these workouts. Why the heck would we want to purposely under-fuel our workouts?

One of the advantageous adaptations of endurance training is that it "teaches" our bodies to better utilize our fat stores as fuel. Remember that even though our bodies store a ridiculous amount of energy in the form of fats, even in skinny people, fats are not easily converted to usable fuel. Since carbohydrate depletion in the form of glycogen is one of the primary limiting factors in endurance sports performance, the better we are at utilizing our fat stores, the longer and faster we can go as athletes. Being able to access and use our fat stores as fuel is a huge positive for the longer distance athlete.

Research has shown that people who have a history of endurance training do in fact burn fat more efficiently than the average person. Some pro triathletes, in an attempt to possibly even better "modify" their fat-burning and fuel utilization capabilities, occasionally engage in longer bike and run training sessions, where they take in significantly less to no fuel at all. The hope is that exercising with decreased carbohydrate stores will force the body to draw upon the fat reserves and potentially become more efficient at doing this over time.

Should you try this? While it is not ideal on a normal basis because training in a low-fuel state could contribute to decreased performance, I actually believe there is some value to engaging in a few of these types of workouts. I wouldn't recommend doing it on a 20-mile (32.2 km) run or 100-mile (161 km) bike ride, but you could try doing a few workouts of a few hours in length on limited fuel and just water. It can also serve to get you even more in tune with your nutritional needs and when exactly you really start to feel the effects of low fueling. Just be sure to properly refuel afterward and for your subsequent workout as well.

I had a client, John, whom I was training for his first Ironman triathlon. We were riding together one weekend, taking part in an organized 100-kilometer (62 mile) bike ride. Even though he was going to do a full Ironman in a little less than a year, John was a relative newbie to the sport, with a few shorter distance triathlons under his belt and a few half Ironman distance races on his schedule in preparation for this race. The bottom line was that John had never paid any attention to his fueling whatsoever, and from my discussions with him, didn't really think it was that important. Even though it was a hot summer day and this ride would be the longest he had ever ridden, he was ready to "wing it" with only a bottle of water.

I decided this was a great chance for him to learn a valuable first-hand lesson about fueling.

You can see where this story is going and ultimately how it will end. Not only did John spend the first few hours of the ride without any real fueling plan at all; he also set out at a pace that was too fast for him at that time.

*Great*, I thought. *Not only is he going to learn about nutrition, he's also going to learn about pacing—the hard way.*

John hammered along for the first few hours, averaging 20-plus miles (32.2 km) per hour up and down the hilly course, a smile on his face throughout. Then, around mile 50, the wheels came off (not literally, of course). Suddenly John went from hammering along to dropping way back, pedaling with his head down, plodding along at 10 miles (16 km) per hour or so. I dropped back and started riding alongside him, explaining to him the concepts of dehydration, fueling, pacing, and more. He learned a valuable lesson that day, one that he didn't want to repeat anytime soon. We began to dial-in his nutritional needs during training and tune-up races, and he went on to have a great race at his first Ironman distance triathlon. To return to our car analogy: If you take a car on a long trip, you need to refuel often or you will run out of gas. Once the car is out of gas, it does not matter how bad you want it to go, it won't. It needs gas, or fuel. The body works similarly; without fuel, it doesn't go. Proper fuel is key to a successful trip, whether it's a vacation or a 100-kilometer bike ride. I use this same analogy frequently throughout the book because it is so simple yet so important to you as an endurance athlete.

Maybe you are still unsure what pre-workout and during workout sports nutrition recommendations are or where you should start. Here are the general rules of thumb; then you can adjust and modify according to your body and what works for you.

**Pre-workout:** Two to four hours prior to workout

- Rich in carbohydrate (bagel, toast, cereal, oatmeal, pasta, rice, potato, fruit, etc.)
- Moderate in protein (lean meat, low-fat dairy, and egg)
- Lower in fat and fiber to prevent gastro-intestinal distress (limit/avoid pastries, white, thick and creamy foods, fried food, extra-high-fiber grains, cruciferous vegetables such as broccoli, cauliflower, Brussels sprouts, etc.)
- Drink 16 to 20 ounces (473.2 to 591.5 ml) water or sports drink

## MY FIRST EXPERIENCE WITH GELS

I was a runner long before I started triathlons, and I vividly remember experimenting with fueling during training for my first few marathons. I was using gels during my long runs and was trying to determine when I should take them and how often. The instructions on the gel pack said to take them every forty-five minutes, so that's initially what I started to do. Over time, however, I realized that I was actually starting to feel light-headed, and my energy level started to drop around forty minutes into a long run. That's pretty early in a run, and I'm sure part of it had to do with improper fueling both day to day as well are pre-workout, but nonetheless, that's when I felt it. I began taking in a gel beginning at thirty minutes and then every thirty minutes thereafter, in an attempt to prevent my body from ever falling behind and feeling negative effects from being under-fueled. That strategy began to work well for me. Soon I was no longer experiencing the same negative physical effects during my longer runs.

Listen to your body during your workouts. It will tell you what it needs. If you are on a fueling schedule and start experiencing consistent drops in energy, try modifying your plan by taking in fuel earlier, more often, more at each interval, or a combination of all three.

**Meal example:** honey wheat bagel with 2 tablespoons (32 g) peanut butter and 1 tablespoon (20 g) honey, one banana, and 16 to 20 ounces (473.2 to 591.5 ml) sports drink **OR** 4 ounces (113.4 g) grilled chicken, 1½ cups (210 g) pasta with marinara sauce, green beans, ½ cup (75 g) chopped fruit, and 16 ounces (473.2 ml) water

**Pre-workout snack:** Thirty minutes to one hour before workout (or right before if training in the morning)

- Rich in carbohydrate (granola bar, dry cereal, bread, crackers, pretzels, or fruit)
- Can, but does not have to contain a little protein or fat (peanut butter, 2 percent string cheese, whey protein in protein bar or drink, lean meat, beef jerky, etc.)
- Drink 5 to 10 ounces (148 to 295.7 ml) water or sports drink

**Snack example:** protein bar OR one banana with 1 tablespoon (16 g) peanut butter

**During workout fueling:**

**General carbohydrate recommendation:** thirty to sixty grams carbohydrate/hour

At first, try breaking carbohydrate up into twenty to twenty-five gram increments (one gel, three to six energy chews depending on brand, a serving of sports beans, half a higher-carbohydrate energy bar, and 5 to 10 ounces [148 to 295.7 ml] sports drink, etc.)

**General fluid recommendation:** 5 to 10 ounces (148 to 296 ml) every fifteen to twenty minutes

- Water is fine during the first hour.
- You need to supplement with carbohydrate and electrolytes after the first hour

or maybe sooner if it is planned to be a long workout or if it is hot and humid outside.

- Setting a timer to vibrate or beep at you can be a good way to "teach" your body how to fuel while training.

## Pre-workout fueling

Fueling is exponentially trickier for triathletes because we have to fuel three totally different sports—swimming, biking, and running. Not only that; when we start doing the longer-distance triathlons, our workouts can run from short thirty-minute sessions all the way up to six hours or more.

You may find your body tolerates pre-workout fueling better or worse depending upon the sport involved. You also may find that certain fueling strategies work better when you are doing long, slow sessions but do not work well when you do hard track workouts or intervals on the bike. Once again, you need to listen to your body and see how it reacts to different workouts and different intensities over time.

## Food journal

Because sports nutrition is so individualized and requires experimentation over time, one of the primary secrets to success is recording what you eat before, during, and after your workouts. This will allow you to see patterns over time and slowly dial-in your best strategies. We often forget what we do when it comes to eating throughout the day, and the same holds true with fueling our exercise. This food journal is a valuable tool to help you gradually put together your perfect triathlon nutrition plan.

It need not be very involved, either. You can record it in the same place you record your workouts, whether that is in a notebook, on your computer, or using a smartphone app. It's actually a good idea to combine the food and workout write-up together because the two are so connected. An entry might look like this:

**SATURDAY 1/4/2013:** 13-mile run. Breakfast @ 7 a.m. ½ cup oatmeal with blueberries, two hard-boiled eggs, one glass of orange juice. 8:30 a.m. Run. Hot. Carried two handheld 20-ounce water bottles filled with sports drink & one gel. Drank every 10 min, took a gel @ 1 hour, felt strong throughout. 2 hrs 10 min. Refueled after with chocolate milk.

The other great thing about keeping a food journal is that it can also help you to lose weight. By chronicling everything you eat all day, you will begin to be amazed at just how much more you consume than you thought, especially while snacking. If you are truly feeding your body optimally every three hours or so, this mindless snacking should be unnecessary. This journal is for your eyes only, so be honest while keeping it, and it will really help you to fuel your body optimally for both your race as well as your life.

Triathlon is indeed a lifestyle, so when we talk about filling the tank and fueling your workouts, what we're really taking about is fueling your life. It may sound corny, but it's true. The more you exercise and train for your triathlon, the more you end up focusing on eating better twenty-four hours a day. Exercise makes you feel better, which, over time, makes you want to eat better as well. Healthy habits do lead to other healthy habits. Give yourself time and make small changes in your diet. Small changes lead to big results when done consistently—and that means better health, a better mood, and a better life.

Proper nutrition is the fourth discipline of triathlon.

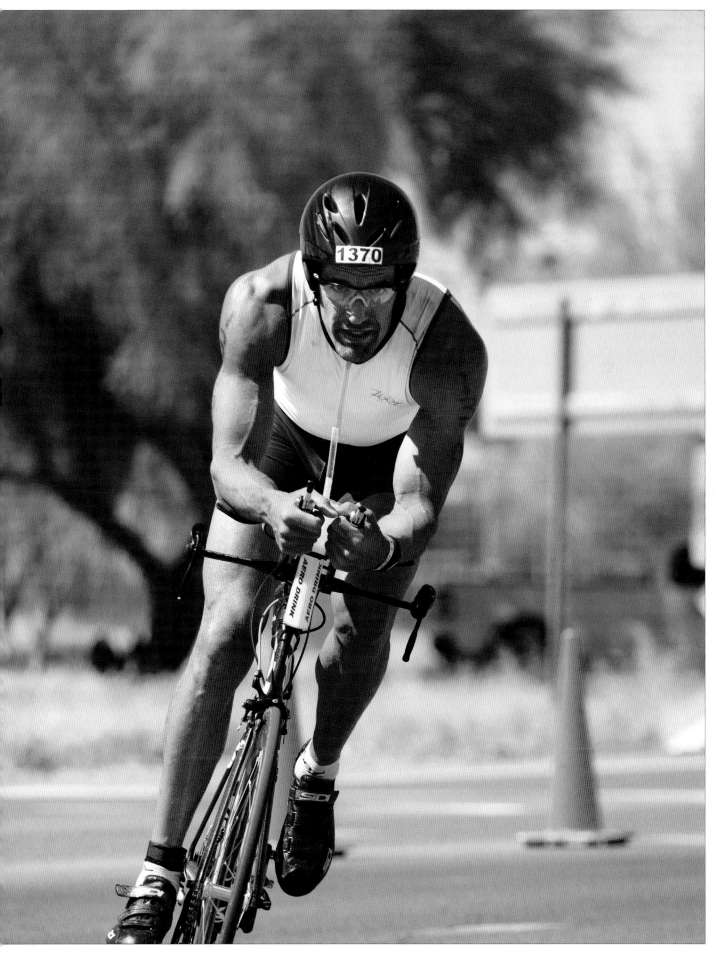

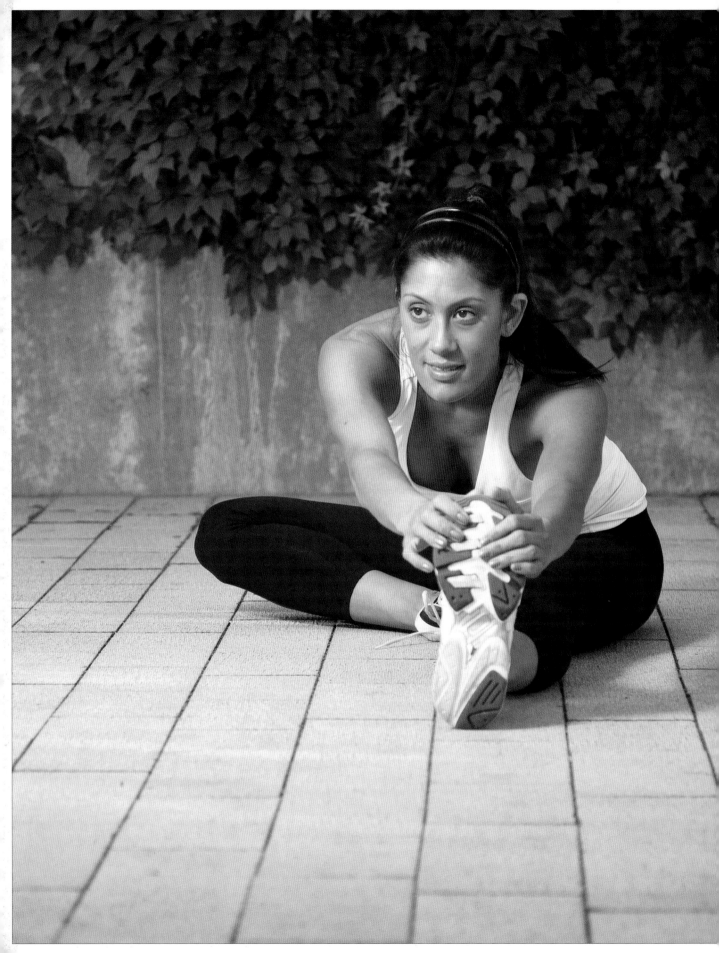

# Refueling: Recovery Nutrition

**ONE OF THE COOLEST THINGS ABOUT** being a triathlete is that we eat a lot of food, and we eat all the time. This serves to perpetually torture our friends and family and is one of the reasons why I truly enjoy the multi-sport lifestyle. Those close to us can't quite fathom how we can be constantly stuffing our faces every time they see us, yet we continue to get fitter and fitter all the while.

We exercise frequently and we have to eat frequently. We are engaging in at least four different exercise modalities, including strength training, and this constant expenditure of energy requires constant fueling. It's not a bad problem to have. It doesn't mean we can eat whatever we want; it means we need to eat good food frequently.

This point bears repeating. As I stated in chapter 7, one of the biggest misconceptions about people who exercise frequently is that "they can eat whatever they want." How great would it be if that were true? It isn't. There is no amount of exercise that can ever offset bad eating habits. It's just that the average person eats pretty well 20 percent of the time and poorly the other 80 percent. They need to reverse those numbers. One of the ways in which we need to change our eating habits for the better is to embrace the concept of refueling after we exercise.

## Weight loss

It's pretty simple. Many people choose not to eat right after a workout for one reason: They want to lose weight. Their thought process is "Why would I want to take in calories right after I worked so hard to work them off?"

Having spent more than twenty years in the fitness industry, I understand why people think this way. When we talk about losing weight, we preach about how it's a simple "calories in and calories out" process. Burn more than you consume each day, and you will lose weight. Then why would we want to ruin what we worked so hard to achieve, taking in calories immediately after we have burned them off?

What you do after your workout is crucial—including what you eat.

It's simple. You're going to take in calories later in the day anyway, but the sooner you take them in, the better. If you work out at 8 a.m., waiting until 12 noon to eat will actually be a detriment rather than a positive. You will not only lose the opportunity to take in your recovery nutrition during the optimal metabolic window of time, but you will also most likely end up eating more throughout the day rather than less as a result of waiting to eat.

Our bodies work optimally when they are fed good food constantly, generally every three hours or so. Waiting until you are ravenous, making poor food choices, and then overeating as well is a recipe for disaster, yet these are common eating habits. When you feed your body a constant mix of high-quality carbohydrates and protein, it hums along like a well-fueled performance vehicle.

## Compensatory eating

You probably know someone who trained for a race such as a marathon or long-distance triathlon, only to have gained weight in the process. They set out with the same goals of so many others; to complete a challenging fitness event and lose weight while doing so. Yet they only achieved one of the two, the former. This phenomenon is known in the fitness world as "compensatory eating." It may sound complex, but it couldn't be simpler: You start exercising more, your appetite grows, you eat more food, and you gain more weight. But it can be avoided. Just as there are a certain

percentage of people who gain weight while training for their fitness event, there are an equal if not greater number of those who show up at the starting line weighing considerably less. Why the difference? Here are the two main reasons why some people pack on the pounds when they should be losing:

1. **They think they can eat whatever they want:** Yes, they buy into the myth about being able to eat whatever you want when you are exercising. Many people who start training for a triathlon or marathon have never exercised that much in their lifetime. They mistakenly believe that they are torching ridiculous amounts of calories during their workouts, and they can therefore eat whatever they want. It's not true. If this were the case, everyone would be swimming, biking, and running. Yes, you can and should eat more food when you are training for your triathlon; you just need to make sure that the vast majority of the time this food is healthy and therefore contains fewer calories than if you binged on junk food. Done correctly, this will put you into a slight negative energy balance each day, which will in turn lead to gradual consistent weight loss over time.

2. **They don't follow a refueling plan:** Of course, you are going to be hungrier when you start training! Why wouldn't you be? You may not be burning as many calories as you or all your friends think you are, but you are in fact expending a large number of calories in your training. You will be hungrier. This is exactly why

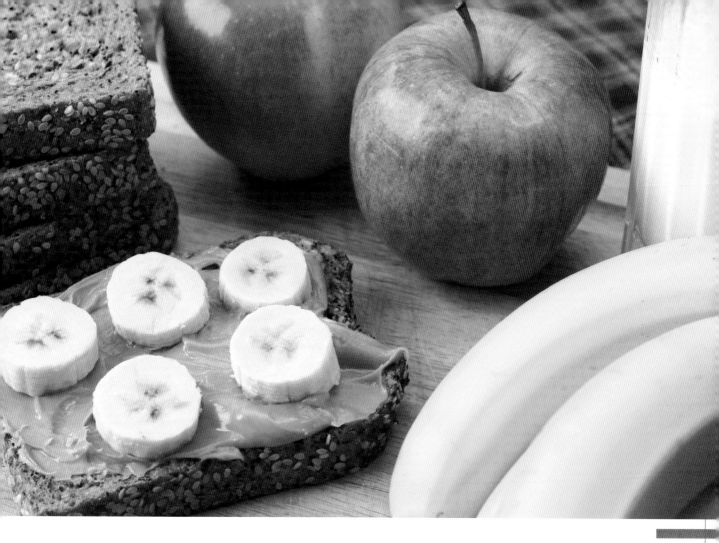

Try to eat healthy carbs with a protein source at every meal.

it is so essential that you implement a smart refueling plan after your workouts, especially the more intense and longer sessions. You need to "re-feed" the body to replace what you have just taken from it. If you wait too long after your workouts to eat again, you will have missed the opportunity to optimally refuel and will most likely make less healthy food choices and eat large quantities due to the fact that you are ravenous.

Most people generally understand the basic concept of fueling up before a workout.

The science of taking in additional calories during the workout itself is a just a little bit more complicated for people to grasp, but even this aspect of sports nutrition is becoming a better understood concept as well. The final piece of the puzzle, refueling after the workout itself, is probably the least understood and therefore the least practiced. Yet it is no less important than fueling before or during a workout, and the more frequently you exercise, the more important refueling becomes.

Refueling equals recovery. In order to get all the essential components of refueling, think of refueling as has having three R's: Replenish, Rebuild, Rehydrate.

Refueling does the following:

1. **Replenish:** Optimally replaces the fuel you burned (carbohydrates) during the workout so you are ready for the next session
2. **Rebuild:** Provides protein to help rebuild the muscles you have broken down during the workout
3. **Rehydrate:** Replaces fluids and electrolytes lost in sweat

As I discussed in the first few chapters on macronutrients, large amounts of exercise deplete our bodies of carbohydrates while tearing apart our muscle fibers, which are made up of proteins. We also lose significant amounts of fluid and valuable electrolytes when we sweat. If we don't replace all of these things constantly and at the optimal times, we will eventually run into problems. Just like we need to have a specific pre-workout and workout nutrition plan in place and implement it each and every session, we also need to have a refueling plan as well. Too many people fail to realize the importance of refueling. I always say that these people have absolutely no idea how great they can feel as well as how much better they can perform. Yes, they can "get away" without refueling after their workouts. But they will pay a price: one they don't realize they are paying, and one that they can avoid by simply taking in food as soon as possible after the workout is completed.

## The metabolic window

*When* you refuel after a workout is just as important as *what* you refuel with. This concept is known as the "metabolic window." Research has shown that there is a certain "window" of time in which the human body is best able to "absorb" and utilize the foods we take in post-workout. Ideally, you want to refuel within thirty minutes or so after your workout is over, but the sooner, the better. It seems that our bodies are simply better able to replenish our carbohydrate stores and utilize the proteins when we consume these foods as close to completing our exercise session as possible. The "metabolic window" is therefore only open for a short amount of time, and we want to take advantage of the benefits that come from refueling during it.

## HOW MUCH?

A simple rule of thumb is to try to refuel with half a gram of carbohydrates per pound of body weight right after your workout. So if you are a 40-year old guy who weighs 150 pounds (68 kg), try to consume seventy-five grams of carbs. How many calories is that?

**75 grams of carbohydrate ×
4 calories per gram = 300 calories**

You also want to take in protein at the same time to help rebuild your muscles as well as to help better absorb carbohydrates, roughly fifteen to twenty-five grams worth.

**20 grams of protein × 4 calories
per gram = 80 calories**

**Example:** ½ scoop whey protein isolate powder mixed in 8 ounces (236.6 ml) low-fat chocolate milk, one large banana, and fifteen grapes

So your post-workout recovery meal might come in at around 380 calories. Again, this is a rough estimate. You might need a little less, or you might even need a little more. You also may be thinking like so many others do—"Wait, that's a lot of food!"

Really? Let's go back to the math. When it comes to discussions about weight, the numbers don't lie, people do!

Using this same 150-pound (68 kg) person as an example, let's say each of his six daily meals is roughly 400 calories:

**6 meals per day × 400 calories**
**= 2,400 calories**

Let's also say he is burning an average of 600 additional calories per day through an hour's worth of exercise:

**2,400 calories energy intake - 600 calories**
**energy expenditure = 1,800 net daily calories**

According to the Institute of Medicine Dietary Reference Intakes report, the Estimated Energy Requirements (EER) for an active 40-year-old male is between 2,800 and 3,000 calories per day in order to maintain energy balance. So this person would be creating a daily deficit of roughly 1,000 calories per day even while eating six meals a day and refueling after workouts. That's two pounds lost per week, without any "dieting" whatsoever. It's pretty awesome.

Here's what a sample 2,400 calorie day might look like, building refueling into the six-meal per day framework:

**Meal #1: 6 a.m.**
250-calorie bagel with 1½ tablespoons (24 g) peanut butter

**Workout #1: 6:30 a.m. to 7:30 a.m.**
6-mile (9.6 km) run

**Meal #2 [Refuel]: 7:45 a.m.**
Half a scoop of whey protein in 12 ounces (355 ml) low-fat chocolate milk, and a banana

**Meal #3 : 11:00 a.m.**
Fifteen whole wheat crackers, 2 ounces (56.7 g) lean meat, one 2 percent string cheese, and 6 ounces (170 g) low-fat Greek yogurt with ½ cup (75 g) berries

**Meal #4: 2:00 p.m.**
One whole wheat pita with 2 ounces (56.7 g) lean meat, ¼ cup (30 g) 2 percent grated cheese, veggies of choice, one-third avocado with a side salad, and one fruit

**Workout #2: 5:30 p.m.**
One hour strength training

**Meal #5 [Refuel]: 7:00 p.m.**
Ready-to-drink post-workout shake with forty to fifty grams carbs and twenty grams protein and 1 cup (225 g) chopped fruit

**Meal #6: 9:00 p.m.**
3 ounces (85 g) lean meat (grilled chicken, fish, or lean beef), 1 cup (140 g) carbohydrate (sweet potato, brown rice, pasta, couscous, or quinoa), and 1 cup (200 g) vegetables or salad

## Simple versus complex carbohydrates

Complex carbohydrates, ones that are less processed and therefore absorbed more slowly, should make up the bulk of our daily carbohydrate intake (bagels, whole wheat bread, oatmeal, pasta, sweet potatoes with skin, brown rice, couscous, quinoa, and whole grain granola bars/crackers/cereal). These carbs are not rapidly absorbed and therefore do not create the sudden spikes in blood sugar and concurrent release of insulin. They provide a steady supply of energy throughout the day without the crash associated with foods containing simple, refined carbohydrates.

As our workout nears, we actually want to switch to the more simple forms of carbohydrates (sports foods such as gels/chews/sports beans, fruit, honey, low-fiber carbohydrates, and the simple sugars found in many pre- and post-workout ready-to-drink shakes), ones that provide our muscles with the most immediate sources of energy. When we exercise, we need fuel and we need it right away, not two hours after we have started our workout or race.

The same holds true with our post-workout carbohydrate intake. We can choose more simple forms to expedite the recovery and restocking process when necessary. I still personally prefer to choose complex carbohydrates at almost all times, except during the race itself when I want that energy to be available as quickly as possible.

## Alcohol

I personally believe in working hard and playing hard. Extremes are easy. It's moderation that is so darn difficult.

I'll never forget going out to dinner years ago with my friend John, an elite triathlete, the night before we were both running the Boston Marathon. We had just ordered our boring pre-race carb dinners, and when the waiter asked what he wanted to drink, he asked for a red wine. This came as a surprise to me—that he would have alcohol the night before a race—but he explained it was a long-standing part of his pre-race "preparation." He went on to have a great race the next day without any negative effects from his alcohol consumption.

Do I recommend drinking the night before a race? Not at all. My point is when you look at the current research, the numerous studies into alcohol's effect on the body post-exercise seem to state the obvious: It's not the best thing after a workout or race. It may impair protein synthesis or the rebuilding of our muscles, it may inhibit the absorption of certain vitamins and minerals, and it cannot be converted to glycogen but is rather converted and stored as fat.

Does this mean you should never drink at all as a triathlete? As I discussed in chapter 7, moderate alcohol consumption does have numerous health benefits, but limiting or eliminating it during training can be a quick, easy way to weight loss. It just means that you may not want to chug a beer right after a workout or a race: Take in your recovery drink or meal, wait a little while, and then celebrate with an adult beverage or two if you so choose.

## Chocolate milk

You may have heard or read that chocolate milk is a great recovery beverage after a workout, and it's true. It may seem counterintuitive, but chocolate milk provides the perfect ratio of carbohydrates to protein, just what our bodies want after a hard exercise session. It seems that from a 4:1 up to a 7:1 ratio of carbs to protein can be the perfect mix to help our bodies repair our muscles and restock our energy stores. So if you have just finished a workout and need a quick recovery beverage, grab a low-fat chocolate milk.

## Real food versus supplements

So what should you use as your recovery nutrition, real food or a store-bought recovery drink or bar? I always say that whenever possible, we should try to eat real food. It's just better for us. Unfortunately, we can't always do that. Sometimes, it's all we have available and/or it's all we can tolerate.

For example, right after a particularly hard track workout or swim session, you might not have a hankering for a big tuna sandwich or bowl of pasta with chicken. Quickly chugging down a store-bought recovery drink or a homemade carbohydrate and protein shake may be all you can literally stomach. It's better to consume something maybe not as natural in lieu of nothing at all.

I am a realist rather than a purist. I have been in the fitness business a long time and realize that there is no "perfect." Do not misunderstand me; I am not giving you an excuse to eat all pre-made sports supplements instead of real food. I am saying that a mix of the two with the majority coming from real food is a great, real-world goal to strive for.

If you are eating five to six meals a day and generally working out one to two times per day, consuming four meals of healthy whole foods and using pre-made recovery drinks after your workout is a pretty good game plan. It's convenient, it's easy, and you know the exact amounts of what you are taking in, which is not generally the case with real food.

I use FRS products, a line of healthy sports nutrition that was originally designed to help fuel chemotherapy patients. They provide me with the simplicity and energy I need when I need it. Drinking a protein shake and eating a banana after a workout is a quick and simple way I ensure that I refuel after certain workouts. I eat real food as well, but sometimes throwing a drink and a piece of fruit in my gym bag is the easiest thing to do.

My best results, for myself and my clients, have always come from attention to the seemingly small things: stretching, sleeping, core exercises, and recovery nutrition.

Refueling after our workouts maximizes the gains from that workout, helps us eat better throughout the day, and prepares us to be at our best for the following workout. Make sure you refuel during the metabolic window, and I guarantee that you'll be amazed at the difference it will make.

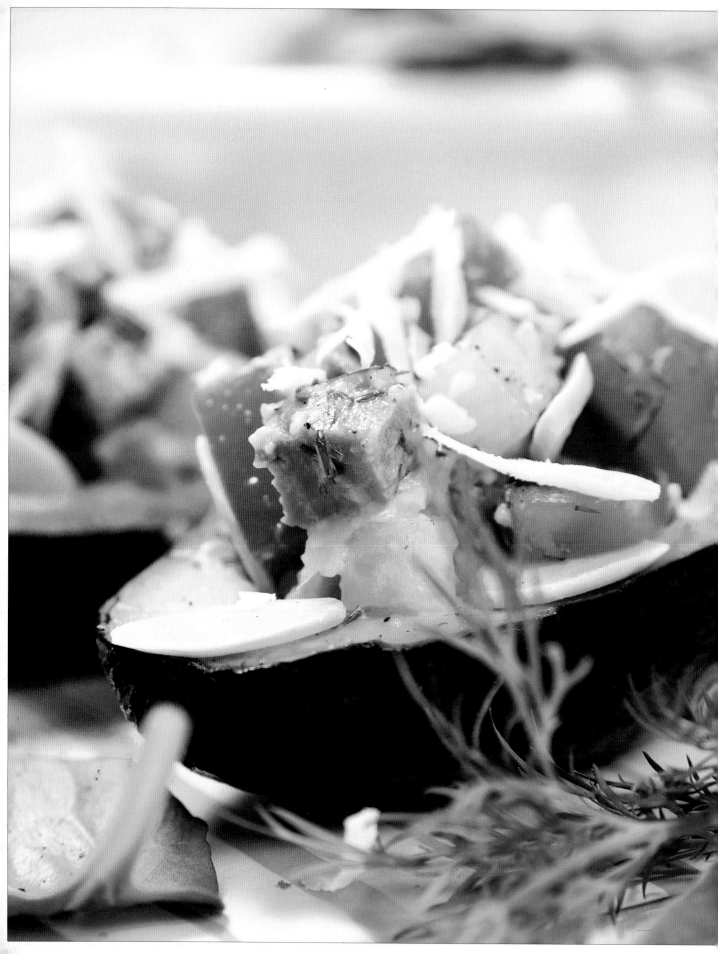

# CHAPTER 10

# Paleo, Vegan, All-Natural, and More: Fueling with Specialty Diets

**LET ME SAY IT RIGHT NOW: I ABSOLUTELY** hate the word "diet." As someone who has spent the better part of two decades in the health and wellness field, I know a thing or two about them, having had hundreds of clients over the years try every conceivable fad diet out there. Simply put, I don't believe in them, and as I discussed in chapter 7 on Dieting Down, the vast majority of diets do much more harm than good.

Why they are harmful bears repeating. When you drastically restrict your calories, often by cutting out whole food groups or types of food, you essentially lose three things: lots of water weight, some fat weight, and even some muscle weight. When you lose the muscle weight, you are in fact lowering your metabolism in the process. That's really not good. So, when you inevitably go off the diet, after starving yourself for weeks on end, and return to eating the same exact amount of food you did before you went on the diet, you will slowly start to gain weight, above what you weighed when you initially started the diet.

You are worse off than if you had never gone on the diet at all.

Yet, since the beginning of time, it seems that man has been on a diet. I wouldn't be surprised if one day we discover that Adam ate Paleo and Eve was pescetarian. We are forever searching for that "magic formula" of foods, or lack thereof, the secret combination that will help us shed those unwanted pounds in record time and keep them off forever.

Low-fat. Low-carbohydrate. Fruit only. Raw only. They all have the same core theme, a food restriction of some kind. Something is "bad," so eliminating it must be "good."

A distinction has to be made here between two different types of "diets." The first type of specialty diet is the one people go on with the primary goal being to lose weight. Think Atkins and South Beach.

Following a special diet? Just make sure you are getting in the right fuel.

The second type is one that people undertake that is a true lifestyle modification, such as vegetarianism and raw food, where the driving force is to improve eating habits and overall well-being. Oftentimes, weight loss is also a goal, but it is not the primary goal. In other words, when the vegetarian hits their weight loss goal, they generally don't start eating meat again.

The waters are a little muddier when it comes to the Paleo- and gluten-free-type diets, which have a combination of the lifestyle modification and losing weight goals, but even though people generally tend to last on them longer than they do the most restrictive fad diets, more often than not, they are not following them years later.

As I stated earlier, my philosophy toward diets is pretty simple. If it has an end date, it's flawed from the beginning. You need to make healthy dietary changes that will ultimately last a lifetime, not a few weeks. If man makes it, try not to eat it. At least try not to eat it frequently.

I also don't subscribe to elimination of whole food groups, unless there is a medical reason for doing so. Extremes are actually much easier than moderation. It's moderation that's really difficult, not avoiding something completely. It's exponentially more difficult to have one cookie a few times a week rather than avoid them completely. For those people who did choose to avoid the cookie completely, that usually means they just replaced it with something else, such as ice cream or the equivalent. We don't quit things: We replace them, oftentimes with something just as bad or, in many cases, even worse.

When it comes to science, current research has shown that it's not the relative percentages of macronutrients that matters when it comes to weight loss; in the end it all comes down to calories. It's calories that count: Calories in versus calories out. Most people don't want to believe it, but that's what the science says. Carbs don't make you fat: It's the amount of carbs you eat that can pack on the pounds. Eat too much protein, and you'll gain weight as well. Any macronutrient (carb, protein, fat) eaten in excess of what you need can add unwanted weight.

Then again, you can also be what is known as "skinny unfit." Sure, you can eat garbage and still be skinny as long as your caloric intake is slightly less than your caloric expenditure. If you take in 1,600 calories of chocolate, processed foods, and other unhealthy fare but burn 1,800 calories per day, you won't gain weight and will in fact lose some over time. You won't have muscle, you won't have the health benefits associated with eating quality foods, and you may not look fit and lean, but what the scale says might make you happy. That's skinny unfit.

Let's cut to the chase. I believe in results. I believe in studying the people who are the best at what you are trying to achieve and emulating them. Science only goes so far; tell me what the best in the game are doing, the ones whose livelihoods depend upon their performances. They are the true "experiments" in the end. What happens in a laboratory, while warranting examination, is of lesser value to me than what is happening on the race course. It's not to say you will look exactly like and/or perform as well as the person you are modeling, but it's likely that you will get close.

So what are the names of the top professional triathletes who follow these "popular" diets? There are none.

The truth is that the vast majority of the best triathletes do not follow any of these plans listed in this chapter. In fact, trying to name even a handful of the best out there today who do is a difficult undertaking. That in and of itself should speak volumes as to the efficacy of these diets for optimal performance in triathlon.

But I am also a realist. Many of you may choose to follow one of these diets for your own specific reasons. You are not professional triathletes. Your livelihood does not depend upon your going top-10 at your next Ironman triathlon. There is no "one-size-fits-all" plan that works for everyone. I am just laying out the facts as they exist today; you can choose to do whatever works for you.

So that's my rant about diets. I get really frustrated with them because I have seen so many people struggle with them, and I know that there is no "winning" with diets, just degrees of losing. Not losing pounds: losing muscle, losing motivation, losing energy, and losing time. I want my clients to get results, not to get frustrated. The only people who truly benefit from diet books are the authors themselves.

What do I eat? A healthy mix of everything: lean meats, fish, healthy fats, fruits, vegetables, and so on; some red wine; some caffeine. Eighty percent of the time, I succeed in eating all of these things in moderation; twenty percent of the time I do not. I am slowly decreasing that twenty percent over time, not because I want to be perfect, but because the more I eat healthy, the less I want anything else. What do I restrict? Processed foods whenever possible. I do my best to eat whole, natural foods, those with as few ingredients as possible. If you had to pin me down to relating how I eat to one specific type, it would be the Mediterranean Diet.

All that being said, many of you may be following some type of diet plan, whether for the short or long term, and I want you to have the best triathlon experience possible, so I'll do my best to inform you so that you can make the best educated decision for you. Here are a few of the more common diets out there and a few quick tips on how you can best fuel your triathlon within the specific parameters involved with each:

**Vegetarian:** It's pretty simple: Don't eat any meat. If it has parents, it's off-limits. Of all the diets listed, vegetarianism and its associated subsets are probably the most popular form of diets followed by some of today's top endurance athletes—some. The list includes ultramarathoner Scott Jurek, elite triathlete Rich Roll, and former pro triathlete Brendan Brazier.

**Modifications:** Being a vegetarian triathlete does not pose significant issues when it comes to fueling. Carbohydrate sources and hydrating are without major restrictions.

The only real issue is when it comes to protein sources in everyday eating, as well as when refueling. Plant protein is not as well absorbed as animal protein, which makes it essential to consume quality and adequate amounts of protein for your body weight and training.

Protein sources:
- Peanut/Almond butter
- Tempeh
- Tofu
- Green peas
- Quinoa
- Beans
- Soy milk
- Seitan
- Hemp seeds
- Edamame

Within the vegetarian category, there are also numerous derivations: Here are a few of the classes of vegetarians.

## FLEXITARIAN

These are people who follow a mostly vegetarian diet but occasionally do eat meat. (Seriously? I'm not counting this one but felt it warranted mentioning because it is out there. I find it ridiculous, analogous to a recovering alcoholic who occasionally drinks. You either eat meat or you don't. Enough said.)

**Pescetarian:** Pescetarians avoid all animal meats except for fish. Fish are high in protein and healthy omega-3 fats, so eating them several times a week can provide huge health benefits.

Healthy fish choices:
- Wild salmon
- Flounder/Sole
- Farmed rainbow trout
- Farmed striped bass
- Canned tuna
- Sardines
- Tilapia

**Modifications:** Again, there's not too much to worry about here as a pescetarian triathlete. Carbohydrates are not an issue. The focus is simply on non-meat protein sources for daily eating and post-workout refueling. Remember that endurance athletes need roughly 0.6 to 0.8 grams of protein per pound (0.5 kg) of body weight. Thus, a 140-pound (63.5 kg) person would need 84 to 112 grams of protein per day, and a 180-pound (81.6 kg) person would need 108 to 144 grams of protein per day.

**Lacto-ovo vegetarian:** They avoid fish, shellfish, and animal meat of any kind, but do eat eggs and dairy. This group is the largest type of vegetarians in North America.

The interesting thing to me about being vegetarian is that, while it does rule out eating meats and in this case fish and other seafood, it doesn't mean you have to necessarily eschew unhealthy options such as processed foods, cookies, cakes, etc. In other words, vegetarian does not necessarily mean healthy. This group still

## LACTO-OVO PROTEIN

- **One medium egg** = six grams protein
- **1 ounce (28.4 g) cheese** = seven grams protein
- **8 ounces (236.6 ml) milk** = eight grams protein
- **6 ounces (170 g) Greek yogurt** = fourteen grams protein
- **½ cup (115 g) cottage cheese** = fifteen grams protein

needs to strive to eat the most natural, whole, unprocessed foods as possible.

**Modifications:** Protein can come from eggs, a phenomenal source, and dairy, which ideally comes from low-fat sources, as well as vegetarian protein powders and milks including soy, hemp, and the like. Eat these protein sources on a daily basis and take in healthy forms of carbs from fruit, vegetables, and whole grains, and you should be able to adequately fuel and refuel your daily activity and training.

**Vegan:** Vegans do not eat any kind of meat, eggs, or dairy products. If it had parents or came from something that had parents, it is a no-no.

Obviously, this group is more restrictive than the others, but the same protein sources outlined earlier for vegetarians are also great options for the vegan.

**Modifications:** Here are the five complete plant-based proteins:

- Quinoa
- Buckwheat
- Hempseed
- Blue-green algae
- Soybeans

Once again, since veganism is more restrictive when it comes to protein sources, the more important concept of fueling with carbohydrates is not the defining issue. We don't fuel our workouts and races with protein, we do it with carbohydrates. However, it is important to get in adequate protein over the course of the day in addition to refueling with carb and protein to help repair any damage done to muscle mass throughout training. Vegan protein powders can also be an easy way to get protein after a workout.

**Raw food:** This group eats only food that is uncooked and unprocessed, such as fruits and vegetables and plant foods in their most natural state. They use dehydrators instead of ovens, keeping the temperature below 115°F to 118°F (46°C to 48°C), believing that high heat robs the food of enzymes and vitamins necessary for proper digestion.

**Examples of raw food choices:**

- Nuts
- Whole grains
- Beans
- Dried fruits
- Seaweed
- Sprouts
- Sprouted seeds

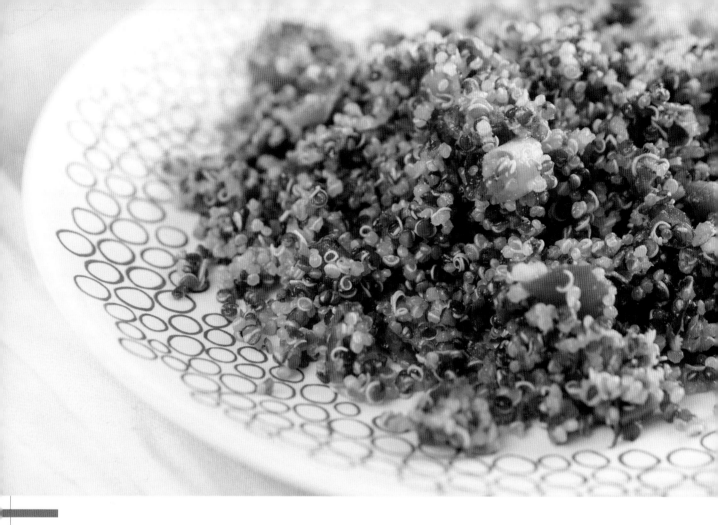

No matter what your diet plan is,
you still need carbs and protein.

**Modifications:** It sounds like the raw food triathlete would have issues adequately fueling themselves, but being able to consume carbohydrate sources such as whole grains, fruits and vegetables, and protein sources such as beans makes it completely fit within the triathlete lifestyle.

**Macrobiotic:** This group consumes only unprocessed vegan foods including whole grains, fruits, vegetables, and sometimes fish. Brown rice and whole grains are staples, and there is an emphasis on the consumption of Asian vegetables, including daikon, sea vegetables such as seaweed, and vegetable-based soups. This diet eschews high-fat foods, most animal products, including dairy products and eggs, and foods that are extremely cold in temperature.

**Modifications:** There are not too many for the macrobiotic triathlete, surprisingly enough. There are great carbohydrate sources to choose from, including whole grains, fruits, and vegetables, and protein sources can come from fish or plant-based options.

**Paleo:** This means to literally eat like a caveman: how our pre-agricultural, hunter-gatherer ancestors ate. Foods would therefore include fish, seafood, and other grass-produced animal products. Fresh fruits and veggies, eggs, nuts and seeds, healthful oils including olive, walnut, and flaxseed are all included in the Paleo diet.

What foods are off-limits? Cereal grains, potatoes, legumes, dairy, and refined sugar. This means no oatmeal, bread, pasta, or beer. Essentially, if it came as a result of agriculture, it is out.

**Modifications:** The issue with the Paleo triathlete lies in the carbohydrate sources. They cannot fuel up with the tried-and-true grains—no oatmeal, no breads. If you are following this diet, then you must get your carbohydrate energy from other sources, such as fruits and vegetables. This could potentially be problematic for the longer-distance triathlete due to the high energy requirements and the limitations regarding carbohydrate sources. Many triathletes need well over 400 grams of carbs per day to fuel all of their training, and many longer distance triathletes likely need well over that amount. Thus, it becomes challenging to get all of that carb from fruits and vegetables alone.

**Gluten-free:** Originally the only medically accepted treatment for celiac disease, this diet is exactly what it sounds like—a diet that excludes foods containing gluten. Most people don't have the faintest idea what gluten is: a combination of two proteins, gliadin and glutenin. Both are found in the endosperm of the wheat, barley, and rye plants. To confuse matters even more, gluten may be added as a stabilizing agent or thickener in products such as ketchup and ice cream, which allows it to appear in hundreds of foods that are not grain based. This diet rules out all ordinary breads, pastas, and many convenience foods.

It is definitely in the category of "fad diets" for those who do not have a medical condition warranting the avoidance of gluten; nevertheless like any other restrictive diet, you will lose weight when following it, and many people swear that excluding gluten makes them feel significantly better.

Many athletes go gluten-free because they believe it eases or eliminates uncomfortable gastrointestinal issues. If that's the case, then more power to them.

However, it is likely that taking gluten out of your diet could lower your daily fiber intake as whole wheat products are typically high in fiber. So taking in adequate fruits, vegetables, and carbs that are high in fiber are essential to promote proper gastrointestinal health.

**Modifications:** Since those going gluten-free cannot get their carbohydrates from the traditional wheat-based breads, pasta, cereals, and the like, they must therefore choose from foods without the gluten for their fueling and energy needs:

- Rice
- Organic corn
- Quinoa
- Potatoes
- Beans
- Fruit
- Vegetables

These are all still great sources of carbohydrates and will optimally fuel the triathlete without consuming gluten.

**Atkins:** The Atkins diet is basically known for one thing: severely restricting carbohydrate intake. It's not concerned with how much you eat but rather what you eat, eliminating refined sugar, milk, white rice, and white flour. Foods such as meat, eggs, cheese, and more are the staples of the Atkins diet; in other words, you're eating almost pure protein and fat.

Having undergone numerous incarnations since it first came out decades ago, the current Atkins diet does allow you to add fruits, vegetables, and whole grain foods after the initial two-week induction period.

**Modifications:** If you have read this book straight through, I'm pretty certain you'll know my take on Atkins. We need carbohydrates to live and to compete. What we don't need are "bad carbs," otherwise known as highly processed carbs, and portions of either good or bad carbs that are too large. That being said, I'm a realist. If you want to follow Atkins for a few weeks as a way to jump-start your weight loss at the very start of your training or, better yet, in the off-season, then so be it. Let me state firmly that it's not how I recommend doing it, but as long as you switch over to eating healthy after a few weeks, it's workable.

**The Zone Diet:** Created by Dr. Barry Sears, this diet proposes a 40 percent carbohydrate, 30 percent protein, and 30 percent fat breakdown to your daily macronutrient intake. It's pretty straightforward.

**Modifications:** The Zone is tough for the triathlete to modify due to the specification of the macronutrient makeup of your diet. It doesn't tell you what you can or cannot eat; it just outlines the relative contribution of each category. For the shorter distance triathlete, I don't see this being much of a problem. For the longer-distance triathlete, however, the rather low 40 percent carbohydrate guideline could be problematic. If you follow the Zone diet and find your energy levels just aren't where you want them to be, you might look into upping your carbohydrate intake, at least during training.

**All-natural**: I have coached several clients who did not subscribe to any of the above diets per se, but rather wanted to eat and drink things that were in the most natural state as possible. This included not consuming certain commercial sports drinks, gels, beans, recovery drinks, and the like.

**Modifications:** The good news is that, in addition to being able to choose from food and drinks in their natural state, there is now a wide variety of all-natural sport supplement products out there as well. One potential problem I have encountered, however, is the use of commercial sports drinks such as Gatorade. Many of those following an all-natural plan do not want to use these types of products. If this is the case for you, I recommend hydrating with water or coconut milk and taking in salt tablets as well if cramping is an issue.

As for options other than the traditional PowerBar, there are now a wide variety of all-natural "energy bars" and similar type products available for those who wish to fuel this way.

There are of course numerous other diets out there today, but these are some of the most popular. What I find incredible is how polar opposite they can be: some focusing on meat, others avoiding it at all costs, yet all sides believe their way is the only way to go. All of these diets have some kind of "scientific evidence" to support their theories.

How can this be so? How can there be so many completely different "perfect" ways of eating?

As I have stated throughout the book and will continue to hammer the concept home, I believe in moderation. It is the hardest thing to do and the hardest thing to sell when it comes to fitness. Extremes are actually easier. Not being able to have something can be significantly less difficult than having a little bit, some of the time. This is especially true when it comes to eating and when it comes to exercise.

All I want for my clients is for them to be as healthy as possible—injury-free and disease-free. Whatever way you choose to eat as a triathlete, remember that it's your health that is paramount. I believe strongly that, as current research shows, healthy, nutrient-rich food contains many disease-fighting properties. We can potentially avoid contracting many of the most common diseases simply by what we eat each and every day. Oftentimes, restricting certain food groups also restricts certain vitamins and minerals that are needed to help our bodies function and fight off disease. Thus, if you choose to follow a diet that eliminates or restricts certain foods or food groups, it is essential that you pay attention to the nutrients you might also be restricting. It's not just about eating less: It's about eating more of what nature has given to us.

So in the end, it doesn't really matter what type of diet you are following as a triathlete. Regardless of the way you choose to fuel yourself, you will always need to focus on the two following things:

1. Taking in enough calories
2. Taking in the right macronutrients (carbohydrates, protein, and fat) at the right times

You need to optimally fuel your body, for your triathlon and for your triathlon lifestyle. That will never change. How you choose to fill up your gas tank is a personal choice. You need to identify what your carbohydrate, protein, and fat choices are within the framework of how you choose to eat, and then fuel yourself before, during, and after exercise with the right amounts and combinations of all three.

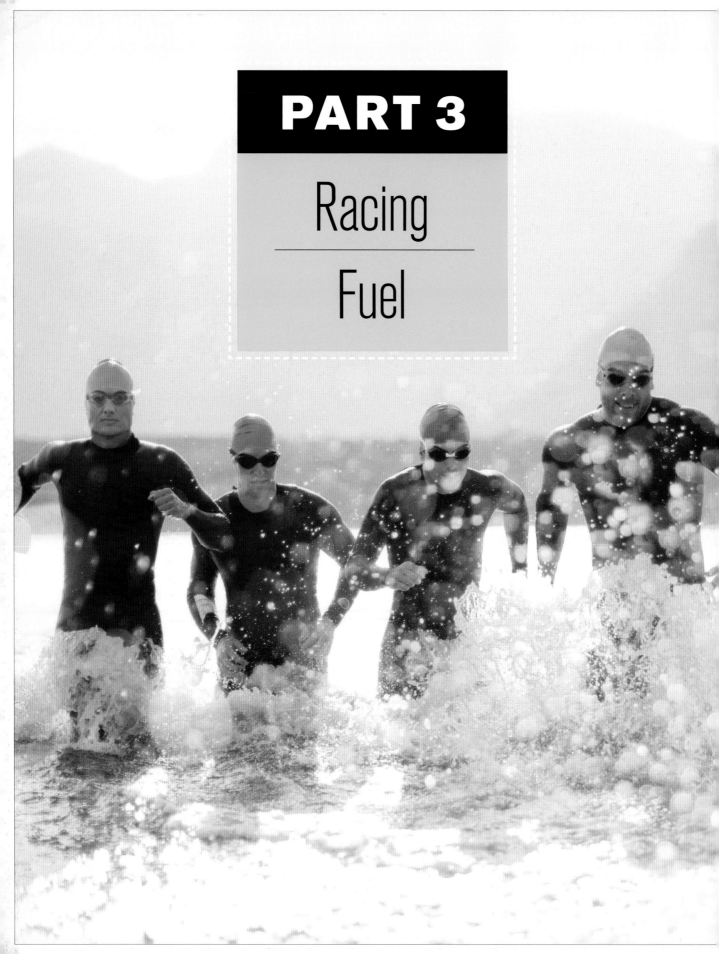

# PART 3

## Racing

## Fuel

# How Do I Carry All This? Race-Day Logistics

# CHAPTER 11

**IF IT'S TRUE THAT MANY TRIATHLETES** leave what they plan on consuming for their nutrition until just before their race, then by definition, they also leave how they plan on getting these calories in until the last minute as well. It may seem like a minor concern, but many find out the hard way that how they carry their race-day nutrition is a crucial component of their success on race day.

During a triathlon, we have two primary times when we can take in fuel, during the bike leg and during the run. As I have said repeatedly throughout the book, the bike leg is the most crucial window of time for us to take in fuel. It gets us through the bike and prepares us for our final leg, the run. That doesn't mean we don't need to take in fluid and fuel during the run, however. The longer our race, the more we will need to take in during the run as well. So we need to formulate a plan during our training concerning exactly how we plan on carrying

our race-day nutrition with us, for the bike as well as the run.

The shorter our triathlons, the less fuel we will need to get us through to the finish line. As we move up in race distance, our energy requirements increase, and we need to figure out how and when we are going to get in the calories necessary to get us through to the end.

When it comes to taking in fuel, one interesting logistical aspect of racing triathlons is that you do have two times during the race when you are not swimming, biking, or running and can use this short window of time to take in fuel—T1 and T2 (transitions 1 and 2). During the shorter races such as the sprint and Olympic distance triathlons, you can fuel up pretty significantly if you choose during these small breaks in the action. For example, if you are doing an Olympic distance triathlon, you can take in a 100-calorie gel and 100 calories of a sports drink in T1, and that will go a long way toward fueling your bike ride, depending on your needs. You might then take in another gel and sports drink in T2 to serve as run fuel.

By race day you should have your hydration and fueling plan ready to go.

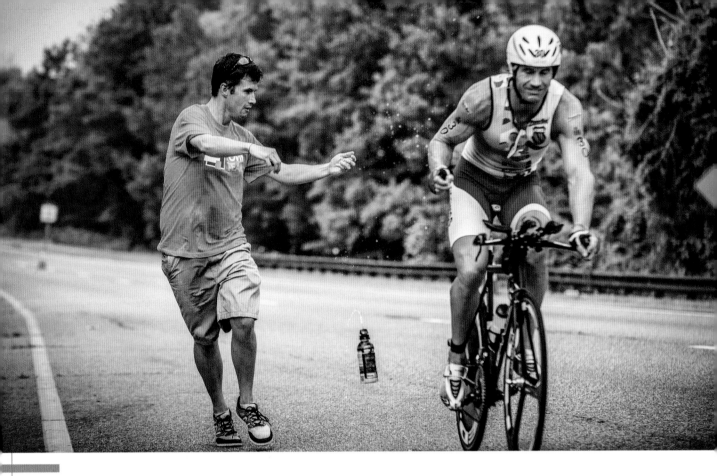

Eating and drinking while biking can be problematic and takes practice.

When you are planning how to carry everything with you during your race, you can lighten the load on your bike and run a bit by utilizing your transitions as fueling stops if you wish. When racing the shorter distance triathlons where your fueling needs might not be as great and/or you want to be competitive and save time in transitions, then you might choose not to fuel up while in T1 and T2. All of these choices come down to your nutritional needs, your goals, and what your preferences are as to carrying fuel with you.

## What about the weight?

I can't talk about carrying nutrition on the bike without discussing what so many triathletes obsess about: excess weight on the bike. Let's be honest: Many triathletes spend thousands and thousands of dollars on their bikes and everything that goes on them to make sure they are as light as can be. They count every gram of weight, from the frame to the pedals to the water bottle cages. The obvious reason is that the lighter the bike, the faster you can go. When it comes to carrying nutrition on the bike, many triathletes think, "Why would I want to weigh down my bike and slow myself down by carrying two extra water bottles with me?"

This makes sense, up to a point. Sure, you don't want to unnecessarily weigh down your bike by taking along a deli's worth of food with you. But you also don't want to limit your fuel and potentially jeopardize your performance just for the sake of keeping your bike as light as possible, especially for the half–Ironman and Ironman distances. There is a balance between keeping your bike light and carrying the necessary amount of fuel with you.

Yes, there will most likely be aid stations along the course, so you can get fuel and fluids from them instead of carrying it with you. Depending upon your race distance and needs, you may choose to carry everything you need with you, you may opt to carry some nutrition with you and supplement with additional energy sources from the aid stations, or you may plan on getting everything you need from the aid stations. Just remember that if you plan on getting everything from the aid stations, you better have practiced using the same brands of nutrition and hydration in training that they will offer on the course, or you could run into trouble.

## THE BIKE

Back to logistics—let's say you decide that your race nutrition plan on the bike involves carrying 1,000 liquid calories of Ensure, four Power Gels, one energy bar, and ten salt tablets; then you plan on supplementing this with additional nutrition from the bike aid stations. How exactly do you plan on physically carrying all of this on the bike? Have you thought about that at all? Maybe you have thought about it and decided how you will do it, but have you practiced doing it? I can't tell you how many times I have spoken to triathletes right before a race, and they are still figuring out the logistics of how they will take in their calories while on the bike. Walk through any race expo, and you will see masses of triathletes scrambling to purchase new means of carrying their nutrition on the bike, things such as aerobar-mounted bottles and Bento boxes, just a day or two before their event. This can be problematic on several levels:

First: If you are purchasing these items just before your race, it means you didn't practice your specific nutrition plan in training. This is not good.

Second: One of the most important rules in triathlon, and any race for that matter, is to never try anything new on race day— nothing. This rule applies to both your nutrition as well as your gear, and in this case, the two are vitally connected.

Let's say you decide to put a brand-new Speedfil in between your aerobars the day before your half–Ironman race. You've never used one before, and now you plan on testing it out for the first time during your race. Leaning forward to drink out of a straw takes practice, especially while biking at high speeds. Also, what are you going to put in the Speedfil? Water? Sports drink? How often are you going to sip from it? How many sips are you going to take when you do? Have you ever practiced taking a bottle from an aid station and then transferring the contents of that bottle to the Speedfil, all while biking?

Or let's say you buy a Bento box to hold your energy bar, a few gels, and some electrolyte tablets. Have you ever practiced taking all these things while actually cycling? Can you physically tear open the energy bar and the gels on the fly? Maybe you plan on taking two electrolyte tablets every hour. What exactly do you plan on putting your electrolyte tablets in? A small plastic bag? A small bottle? Can you open either of these while biking? And you can't just throw the garbage on the road, either. That is grounds for disqualification in most races, so you also need to be able to put the wrappers in your jersey pockets, Bento box, etc. These questions may not seem like a big deal, but they are crucial. If you can't get to your race nutrition and supplements during your race, what good are they?

Finally, attaching anything new to your bike before a race means that this equipment has not been road-tested. It's a rule of life as well as triathlon that things can and will go wrong. This new equipment can be improperly mounted, rattling around or worse yet coming loose in the middle of your race. If this new piece is holding the majority of your race nutrition and it flies off at mile ten of your Ironman, you're in trouble. One loose screw can put an end to your race.

There are three basic places you will get your calories from during the bike leg of your triathlon: On your person, on the bike itself, and from the aid stations.

**On your person:** You have the option of wearing a race jersey with pockets during your tri. These pockets can be a great place to carry nutrition such as a few bars and gels and supplements such as your electrolyte tablets while on the bike. Jersey pockets provide relatively easy access and do not pose the potential problems of bike-mounted storage. Many triathletes use these pockets during their training, thus it is a good idea to continue to do so during their race.

## WHAT NOT TO DO

I have made every possible mistake during my 21 Ironman races and countless shorter distance triathlons around the world, including putting new equipment on my bike right before the race. This included replacing my two seat-mounted water bottle holders with new super-expensive ridiculously light carbon ones before a half–Ironman race. Super-light as they may have been, they also functioned more like silent mortars than water bottle holders, launching the majority of my nutrition when I hit the first little bump in the road. Trust me; you never want to reach back for your primary race calories only to realize that they have magically disappeared.

The author taking salt tablets during an especially hot Ironman Kentucky.

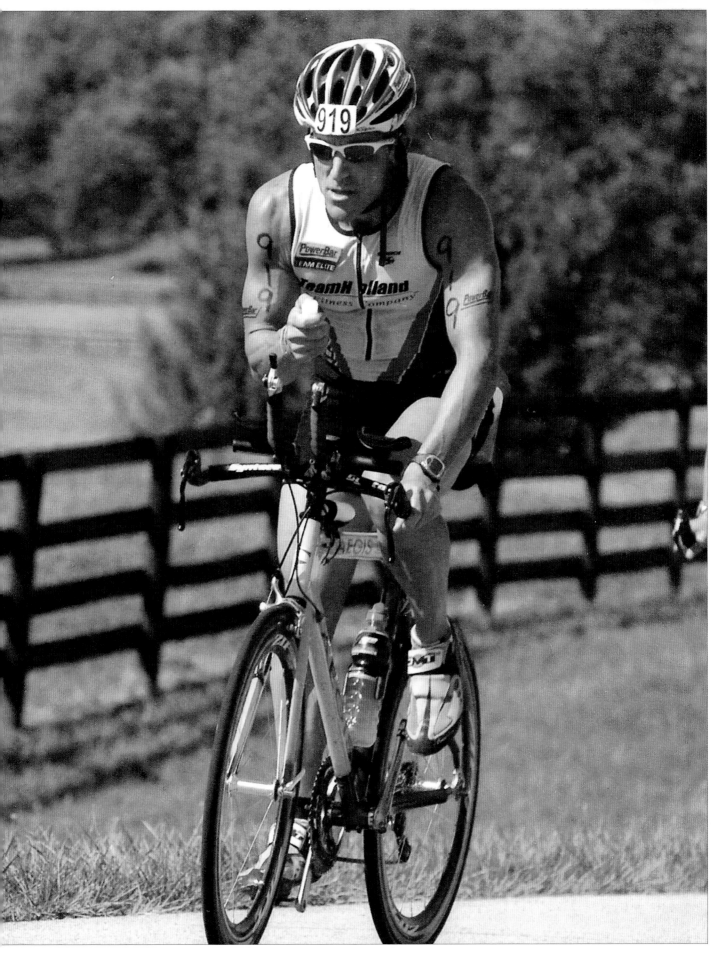

Like everything you choose to do during your race, using jersey pockets to store your nutrition comes down to personal preference. I've seen triathletes stuff these pockets to near overflowing, while others prefer not to use them at all. I will repeat this over and over throughout this book because it is so vitally important: What you choose to do during your race, you should have practiced in your training. If you've never utilized your jersey pockets before, doing so on race day can be problematic. Things can fall out, they can rub you the wrong way and chafe, and/or the feeling of having these items on your back can just downright annoy you if you're not accustomed it, especially during a long race.

**On the bike:** There are so many options today for how and where you can carry your nutrition while on the bike. One or two years from now, there will be even more as the equipment manufacturers in the sport are constantly innovating and improving this technology.

The most basic method is the simple water bottle cage, attached either to the bike frame or to the seat. It depends on your specific brand of bike, but many bikes can have one or two water bottle cages on the frame and two can be mounted behind your seat. You can also have a bottle on your aerobars, either lying horizontally or vertically with a straw attached. You can use the bottles to hold fluids for hydration, calories in the form of liquid nutrition, or both.

The Bento Box is another way in which to carry nutrition and other items with you on the bike. They vary widely in size, materials and design, but are essentially small bags that attach to your bike frame and can be used to carry gels, energy bars, electrolyte tablets, or anything you want to cram in there. Just remember that whatever you do put in your Bento Box, you will have to be able to open and consume while cycling in a race situation. Be sure to practice your Bento Box fueling strategy in training.

**The aid stations:** Aid stations can offer as little as water in some smaller, shorter triathlons to the veritable smorgasbord found during most Ironman distance events. Energy gels, energy bars, bananas, water, sports drink, soda—these are but a few of the offerings on triathlon race courses. Your plan should be to determine what will be offered during your specific triathlon, which can often be done by looking on the event website, and then using these products in training, right down to the specific brand and flavor. Determine as soon as possible what works and what does not and then design your race nutrition strategy accordingly.

## THE RUN

The rules that apply to carrying fuel during the bike leg also apply to the run. You need to be able to answer the same questions as early on in your training as possible. What is your nutrition plan for the run leg of your triathlon? How and what do you plan on carrying with you? What will you get from the aid stations? Just like the bike, the sooner you can dial this all in during training, the better.

If I sound like a broken record about figuring out what works for you nutritionally while in training, it's because it is that important. Don't wait until it is too late to plan your run fueling, or you'll jeopardize all the hard training you put in for your triathlon. It is the final leg of the triathlon, and if things are going to fall apart, it's most likely to happen while you are on that run course. Need proof? Just watch the final miles of any Ironman distance triathlon.

The shorter your triathlon, the less fuel you need to carry with you. If your race is going to have particularly well-stocked aid stations on the run, this may also decrease your need to weigh yourself down with extra calorie-containing gear. But realize that you should never rely on the aid stations to have exactly what they say they will have. They can and do often run out of products, especially if you are coming through later in the race, so the more you can bring with you, the better. You have to determine what you used in training and what you will want on race day. For example, you may be doing an Olympic-distance triathlon. You drank orange Gatorade while on your runs in training, and it worked really well for you. If they won't be offering it on the race course and you want it, you will have to formulate a plan for carrying it with you. There are two main ways triathletes generally carry fluids and fuel with them while on the run:

1. Around the waist with a running belt: Like Bento Boxes, these fueling belts vary widely in design. Their purpose is to carry your fluids as well as little extras such as gels and electrolyte tablets around your waist while you run. The number and size of bottles they carry varies widely as well, from one small bottle to half a dozen or more. They are often called Fuel Belts, which is actually a specific brand and one of the more popular types of nutrition belts. Of these types of belts, one of the more popular versions has four small bottles and one pouch to carry extra gels, salt tablets, etc.

2. In their hands: While a less-popular method than carrying fluid and fuel around the waist, there are many different products available that allow a triathlete to carry nutrition attached to their hands if they so choose. These "handhelds" can also have different sizes of bottles along with pockets to hold things such as gels, blocks, and salt tablets.

One of the concerns triathletes have with using things such as a nutrition belt or handheld water bottle is that their running form will be compromised and/or it will "weigh them down." This is a valid concern and yet another reason why you should try out any new method in training before you use it in a race. These belts and handhelds have come a long way and are designed to be as unobtrusive as possible. Also, just look at the pros: Many utilize some form of self-contained fueling system while running, especially the longer distance triathlons, and it's not just because they are sponsored by those companies. They know what has worked for them in training and also the importance of adequately fueling their run.

## IRONMAN GERMANY

Ironman Germany was my second Ironman –distance race way back in 1999. I wore a four-bottle Fuel Belt, each bottle filled with two gels, premixed with a sports drink. So eight gels in total, and I was ready to take in one gel every thirty minutes by drinking half a bottle. I had used this technique in my first Ironman and even several prior marathons. When I crossed the finish line in Roth, the bottles were all full. I hadn't used them; I had chosen to grab nutrition from the aid stations instead.

My point is that it didn't bother me one bit to wear the belt. I barely felt it during the run. The nutrition I carried with me ended up serving as insurance; it was there if I needed it, but I ended up not needing it. It didn't slow me down, and I had a great second Ironman experience. I no longer use the belt today, but it served me well when I did.

Let's be honest, a big part of the fun of triathlon is in all the great gear we can buy for the sport. Part of this gear includes a variety of methods for carrying nutrition while biking and running. Your job is to do a little research. Start searching the Web, talk to your triathlete friends, flip through your tri magazines, and ask at your local bike shop. Just like choosing a bike, what types of equipment you choose to carry your nutrition is varied and ultimately a personal choice. Just make your decisions as soon as possible after you decide to start training for your race and then practice implementing them into your training every chance you get. Remember, no matter how solid your nutrition plan, it only works if you actually can physically bring it with you and take it in on race day!

You can carry your fuel with you, use the aid stations, or both.

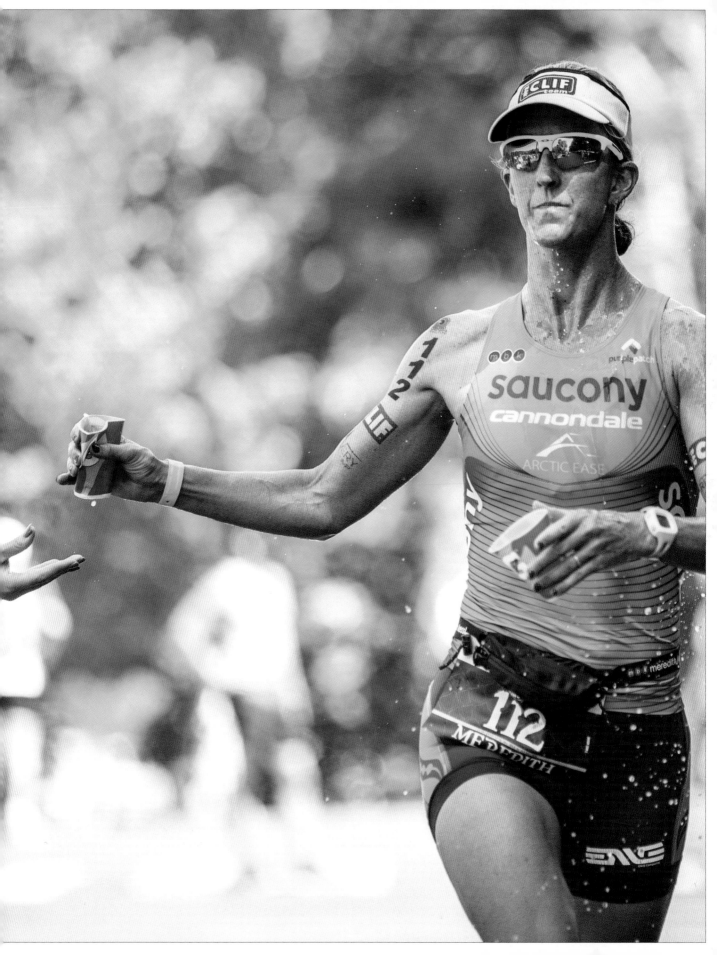

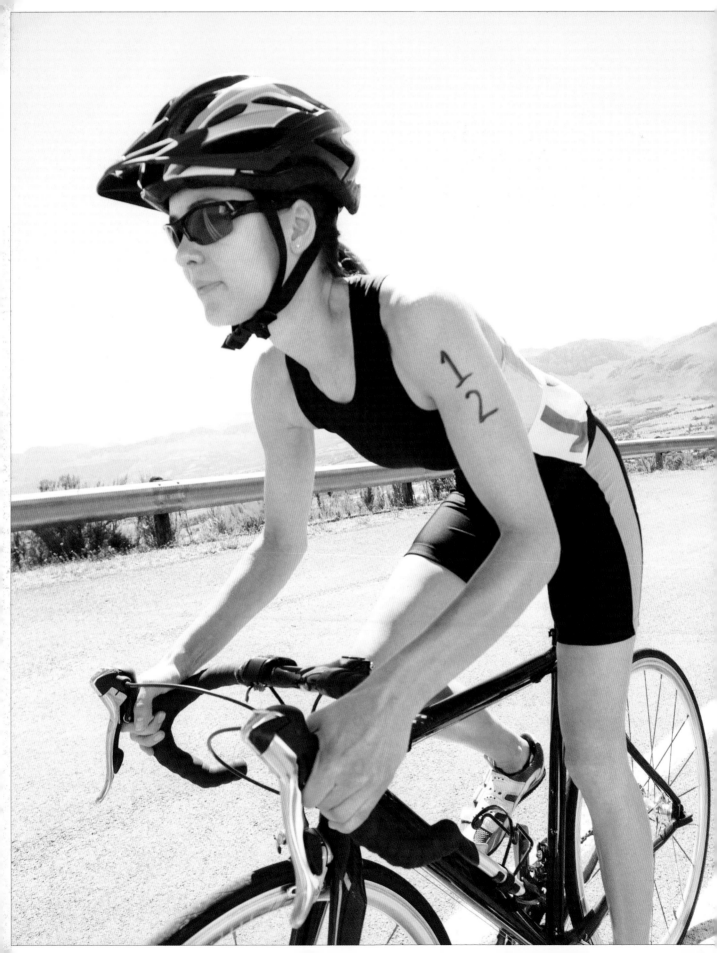

# Fueling Your Sprint Triathlon

# CHAPTER 12

**THE SPRINT-DISTANCE TRIATHLON IS** the shortest of the four standard triathlon distances. It is also the only distance triathlon that can vary slightly in the length of the swim, bike, and run legs; however, the distances below are generally accepted for the sprint:

**Swim:** 0.5 miles or 750 meters

**Bike:** 12.4 miles or 20 kilometers

**Run:** 3.1 miles or 5 kilometers

Again, races described as being "sprint" triathlons can be slightly longer or shorter than the distances above.

Using those standard distances for each leg, the top racers will generally finish in around an hour, while the last few will come in around an hour and forty-five minutes or more.

Given the relatively short duration of a sprint triathlon, your nutritional needs during the race itself are not very high. Most people can exercise for an hour without taking in additional energy. Remember, our bodies store roughly 2,000 calories

The shorter your race distance, the less your fuel requirements.

worth of energy in the form of glycogen in our muscles and liver. If the average person burns roughly 600 calories per hour while exercising, and our fuel stores are topped off before our sprint tri, then we should be able perform well on our fuel stores alone.

So pre-race fueling is important when it comes to fueling the sprint triathlon. Now this does not mean that we need to "carb up" as we would for longer races. It simply means we want to make sure our fuel stores are full to almost full.

## Pre-race jitters and gastrointestinal distress

The sprint is quite often a person's first triathlon. The first-time race jitters and subsequent stress can manifest itself in stomach aches, stomach cramps, and even, yes, diarrhea. Eating during this time of stress can therefore add to this physical discomfort. Because the nutritional needs of the sprint triathlon are not extremely great due to the short workout time, I believe that many sprint triathletes, especially first-time

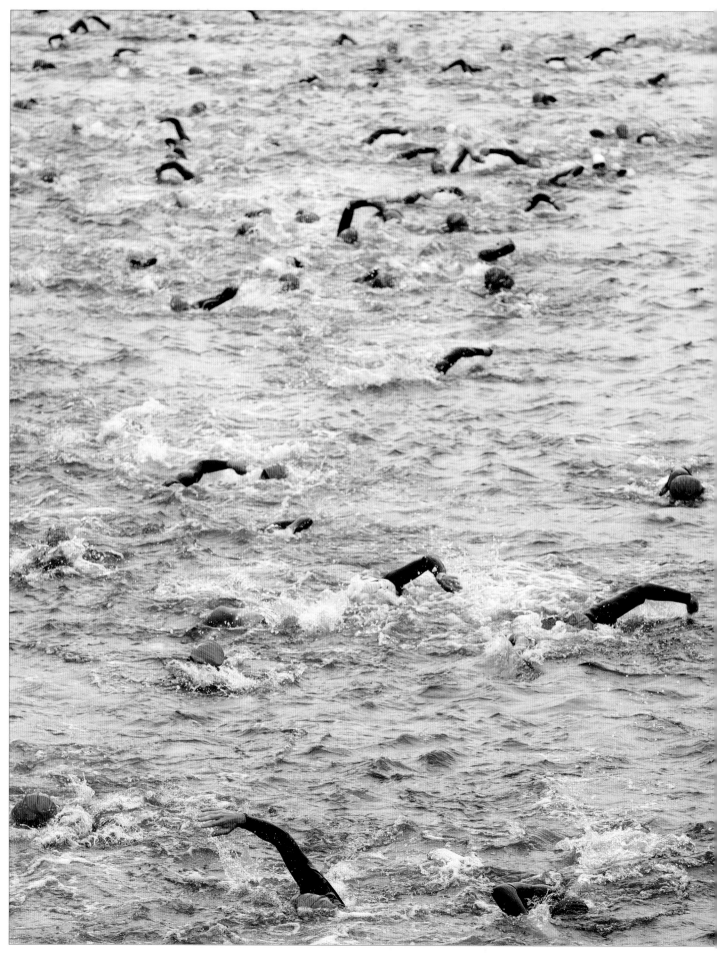

triathletes, are better off eating less rather than more during the race, especially just before the race start. Here are the basic guidelines for fueling your sprint distance triathlon:

## The day before your race

Carbohydrate loading: Again, since the race is roughly one to two hours in duration, no significant carbohydrate loading plan is necessary. Eat as you normally do the day before the race, making sure not to take in any food or liquid that you are not extremely accustomed to. As with your standard day-to-day diet, you should try to eat quality carbohydrates and protein at each meal. You may want to eat your dinner a little earlier than normal to give your body some extra time to process the food before your race. Dinner should be a simple meal of carbohydrates and protein, such as pasta with chicken.

Hydration: There is no need to hydrate excessively the day before your race. As you will most likely be taking the day off or just doing a quick "shake-out" workout of 15 to 20 minutes or so, you will not be sweating and thus in need of taking in more fluid than normal. Aim to drink half of your body weight in water in ounces, spreading out the fluid intake throughout the day.

Try to eat breakfast a couple hours before the race starts to give your body plenty of time to process the food.

## Race morning

Your pre-race dinner and breakfast should supply you with almost all the calories you need to get you through your sprint triathlon.

Your pre-race breakfast should be something simple and something you are extremely accustomed to eating. Ideally, you are consuming a complex carbohydrate for sustained energy and protein or some

### FIVE PRE-RACE BREAKFAST EXAMPLES

1. English muffin with 1 tablespoon (16 g) peanut butter, ½ cup (75 g) berries, 8 ounces (236.6 ml) water, and 8 ounces (236.6 ml) sports drink

2. ½ cup (40 g) oatmeal (measured dry) with 1 tablespoon (20 g) honey, 2 egg whites, 8 ounces (236.6 ml) water, and 8 ounces (236.6 ml) sports drink

3. 6 ounces (170 g) low-fat Greek yogurt (if dairy pre-workout does not bother you) with ⅓ cup (27 g) granola, 8 ounces (236.6 ml) water, and 8 ounces (236.6 ml) sports drink

4. 1 whole wheat waffle toasted with 1 tablespoon (16 g) almond butter, 1 fruit, 8 ounces (236.6 ml) water, and 8 ounces (236.6 ml) sports drink

5. Finicky stomach: 150- to 250-calorie protein bar, 8 ounces (236.6 ml) water, and 8 ounces (236.6 ml) sports drink

healthy fat to stabilize your blood sugar. You also want to give your body plenty of time to process this food so it's not sitting heavy in your stomach when the starting gun goes off, so you want to try to eat breakfast two hours or so before the race if possible. Some races start at 6 or 7 a.m., so eating several hours before the race would mean you need to get up pretty early. The good thing about triathlons is that you are most likely getting up early anyway to get all your stuff together and get down to the race start, so try to eat right after your alarm clock goes off. Don't wait to eat, even if you're not hungry.

You can sip on water in the hours leading up to your race, but don't overdo it. Fifteen to twenty minutes before your swim start, you could drink 10 ounces (295.7 ml) of a sports drink or take in one energy gel if you feel you need extra energy at the start.

## T1

You will exit the swim and run to the transition area you have set up that morning. This will be your first opportunity to fuel yourself during the race itself. Once again, the sprint triathlon is relatively short, so you by no means need to overdo fueling at this point, and many will opt not to fuel at all. This is, however, a good chance to hydrate because the body does lose some fluid from sweating during swimming, especially if you're wearing a wetsuit and/or it is a hot morning. As always, I would recommend choosing a sports drink over water in order to get a little extra energy in the form of

calories and electrolytes. Eight to 10 ounces (236.6 to 295.7 ml) or roughly half a normal size bottle should be plenty for most.

If you are someone who thinks they need additional calories during the race, or you weren't able to eat as much pre-race, this first transition can be a great place to take them in. It only takes a few seconds to take in a gel or part of an energy bar during transition, and you don't have to worry about doing so while moving on your bike when it can be difficult. This especially holds true for first-time triathletes. Biking while eating and drinking can be tricky for those newer to the sport. Crashes and falls do often occur when people unaccustomed to it try to take in fuel and cycle at the same time. So if you have any reservations about hydrating or eating while on the bike, front-load your fluid and fuel while in T1.

So, quick tips for T1:

- 8 to 10 ounces (236.6 to 295.7 ml) of fluid, preferably a sports drink
- 100 to 150 calories in the form of an energy gel or another semisolid source if you feel you need additional fuel

## The bike leg

The bike leg of most sprint triathlons is around 12 miles (19.3 km) long, so the faster riders can do it in thirty minutes or less, and the average riders will take a little under an hour, depending on the course and conditions. You still have to run when you get off the bike as well, usually another 3 miles (4.8 km), which can mean another twenty to thirty minutes or more of exercise.

One of the most important rules about triathlon is that "The bike sets up the run." This applies to pacing as well as fueling. Both are important concepts, yet rarely followed. If you push the bike too hard when it comes to pace, your run will suffer. If you under-fuel while on the bike, your run will suffer as well.

The good news for sprint triathletes is that the shorter the race distance, the less crucial both of these concepts become. It doesn't mean they're not important; it just means you can get away with both a little bit more because you don't have as far to go.

When it comes to fueling on the bike, there are two important questions you will have answered long before racing your sprint triathlon. One is, will there be aid stations on the bike? And two, will I be taking any fluid or fuel from these stations themselves?

I believe in being as self-contained as possible regardless of the race distance. This means bringing as much of my fluid and fuel as possible on the bike itself. Now, the longer the race distance, the less able we are to do this as triathletes, especially when it comes to fluid replacement. When it comes to all our major sources of calories, however, we can have the vast majority of them on our bike at the race start.

I also believe one of the easiest fueling strategies for the sprint triathlete while on the bike is to take in a sports drink. It provides fluid replacement, electrolyte replacement, and additional calories as well. Having one bottle filled with a sports drink on the bike can provide everything

you need to fuel the bike leg of your sprint triathlon while setting you up for a great run. The fluid is also the easiest fuel for your body to absorb, much easier than semisolid or solid foods. The physical act of taking solid foods on the bike can also be problematic, such as opening an energy bar while cycling; for many, another reason why getting in your fuel from a bike bottle can be exponentially easier.

Don't misunderstand me; some of you may still prefer to take in a gel or bar while on the bike. This comes down to personal preference and what you feel you need, having experimented with these things during your training. Just know that the denser the fuel you ingest while on the bike, the more it can affect you negatively during your run.

## T2

So now you have made it through the swim and you survived the bike leg. You're back at T2 and ready to head out on the run. If you have followed a smart fueling plan up until this point, starting with your dinner the night before, your pre-race breakfast, and your fueling while on the bike, there's not a lot left to do when it comes to fueling up. Frontloading your fuel is an important concept because the run leg is when your body least wants to take in calories. Your body is supported while on the bike, and this reduces the amount of negative gastrointestinal effects that fueling can have on the body. By the time you get to T2, hopefully all you have left to do is hydrate, if anything at all.

Just like in T1, you may want to take in 8 to 10 ounces (236.6 to 295.7 ml) of fluid while in T2. If you feel you will need additional calories and/or additional electrolytes, choose a sports drink.

T2 is not the place you want to eat or drink too much and then go out on the run feeling bloated. Making the transition from biking to running is difficult enough for most. Add in gastrointestinal distress, and you're setting the stage for a less than enjoyable finish to your race. The faster you plan on running, the less likely you will be to fuel up while in T2. If you are trying to run six- or seven-minute miles (1.6 km), there is not much race left. You don't need much fuel to get to the finish line. Your body also won't be too happy about trying to digest anything while you run at a high intensity.

If you are planning on running 10-minute miles (1.6 km) or more, you may want a little extra "boost" to get you through to the end. It may be more psychological than physical, but whatever the reason, do what works for you.

Here is a quick nutritional race report from my client Nicole, who was participating in her second sprint-distance triathlon:

•••

*I had a quick carb/protein shake when I woke up, then a gel thirty minutes before the swim. I brought a bottle of Gatorade on the bike and drank half on the way out and half on the way back as you suggested. It was hot, so it was easy to drink, and it helped. Chugging down the second gel before the run can be gross, but I always feel that I need the boost. You know me, I love my morning coffee. The race was so early that I had to miss it. So I used the caffeinated gels. Not the same, but mentally, it does the trick.*

•••

Nicole's report is a great example of how your fueling strategy can be a combination of the mental and physical. She most likely didn't need the final gel to get her through the run energy-wise, but if it served to provide the mental "boost" as she described, then it was an invaluable part of her race-day plan.

So fueling your sprint-distance triathlon comes down to just that: Combining what your body needs with what you think you need. The energy requirements are not great given the relatively short exercise time, but triathletes, especially first-timers, will often take in a bar, gel, or the like for the psychological benefit more than the physical need.

## Quick notes for fueling your sprint triathlon

- There's no need to carbohydrate load.
- Breakfast should be something simple and something you commonly eat.
- Proper hydration is your primary focus during the race, but dehydration should not be a major concern given the shorter workout time.
- "Bonking" should not be an issue.
- If you have eaten a good pre-race dinner and breakfast, your fuel stores should be high enough to get you to the finish line.
- If you want to take in calories during the race, take liquid and semisolid forms.
- And most of all, do what has worked for you in training.

For many of you, a sprint-distance triathlon will be your first. I encourage you to make these your three primary goals:

1. To finish
2. To have fun
3. To want to do it again

If you hit all three of those goals, your race has been a huge success, regardless of your finishing time. Proper nutrition will help you achieve all three.

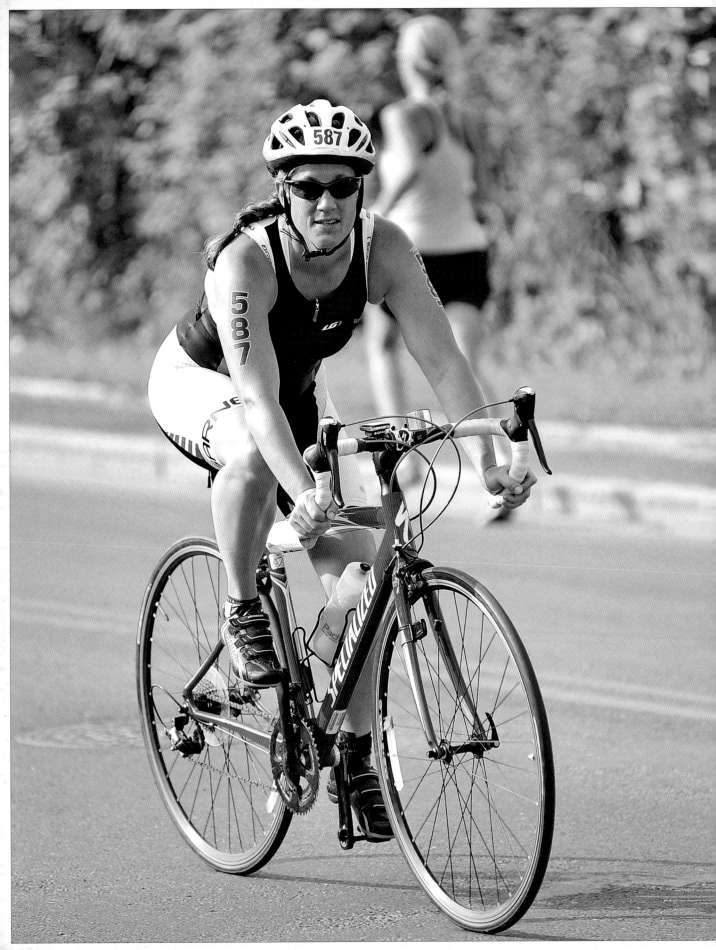

# Fueling Your Olympic Distance Triathlon

**THE OLYMPIC DISTANCE TRIATHLON IS** the perfect triathlon for many. The distances involved are not too easy yet not too hard, a perfect challenge and fitness goal. The training involved does not require a huge time commitment and will therefore not dramatically impact your day-to-day life.

Unlike the sprint distance triathlon, where there is often variability in the length of each leg, Olympic distance triathlons are always the same: A swim of 1.5 kilometers (1 mile), a 40 kilometer (25 miles) bike, and a run of 10 kilometers (6.2 miles). The average times for each discipline vary relative to numerous factors, but forced to use basic round numbers, average swim times would be around thirty minutes, bike times would come in a little under ninety minutes, and run times would average just under an hour. In total, the average Olympic distance triathlete would finish the race in the neighborhood of three hours. That's three hours of continuous exercise.

The more your work on your fueling in training, the more you will enjoy your race.

That's considerably longer than the casual long workout most people would engage in at the gym or while exercising outdoors. Sprint triathlons generally take just over an hour for many to complete, and therefore the fueling requirements are considerably less than that of the Olympic. You may have a few sprint triathlons under your belt already. You may have paid close attention to your fueling plan during these races, or you may have just "winged it" as many first-time triathletes do and pretty much just made it up as you went along. Though you can get away with less attention to your fueling plan in sprint triathlons, the requirements of racing the Olympic distance can be much less forgiving.

Many triathletes are runners first, having completed numerous races of various distances, from the 5 kilometer (3 mile) up to the half marathon or marathon. You may fall into this category as well. For those who have run a 10-kilometer (6.2 mile) race, which takes around an hour for the average runner to complete, you know what it is like to race for roughly the amount of time it takes to complete a sprint distance triathlon.

You may have hydrated during those 6.2-mile (10 km) running races, or maybe not. Most people do not take in any semi-solid or solid foods during these races because the energy requirements do not call for it. Using these running races as a comparison, you can see how hydration is the primary focus within the race when it comes to the sprint distance tri.

Using this same type of comparison, let's look at the half marathon running race distance versus the Olympic triathlon. If we use ten minutes per mile (1.6 km) as the average speed of half marathoners, then finishing times would come in at 130 minutes or a little over two hours. So to put it into perspective, this would be almost an hour less than the average finishing time for an Olympic triathlon.

Many runners realize that they cannot simply "wing it" when running a half marathon. They eat a little more the night before their race and pay a little extra attention to what they eat on race morning. They hydrate along the course at the aid stations and perhaps even take in extra calories in the form of a gel or sports beans along the course as well. Some may even choose to bring extra fluids and food with them, carrying the fuel by means of a race belt or other similar device.

If the aforementioned are required for a half marathon race, then fueling an Olympic triathlon, which takes even longer to complete, requires even more when it comes to fueling. The last thing you want to have happen is to train hard for your Olympic tri and to not enjoy the race due to a poor fueling strategy.

Even though the Olympic distance triathlon may require two to three hours or more of continuous exercise, we have to remember that the body can store roughly two thousand calories worth of glycogen. Using the same 600-calorie per hour average energy usage number, you can see that the energy requirements for this distance should still generally not exceed our stores if we begin the race with a full tank.

Still, two to three hours is a decent amount of time to push our bodies in a race. Dehydration is definitely a possibility, much more so than in a sprint triathlon, especially when racing in hot and humid climates. So when it comes to the Olympic distance triathlon, we need to make sure we are fueled up fully beforehand, possibly take in additional calories during the race, and hydrate adequately during the bike and the run.

## The day before your race

Carbohydrate loading: While two to three hours of exercise is not just a "walk in the park" for most, there is no need to significantly alter your daily eating habits, provided they are good habits. You can choose to add some extra carbohydrates to each meal the day before, but do not overdo it. If you are only going to take in additional carbs at any one meal, then it should be your dinner. Once again, everything you eat the day before should be foods that you are accustomed to eating. This is not the time to try Indian food for the first time or experiment with a new restaurant the night before. Keep your meals simple, avoid foods high

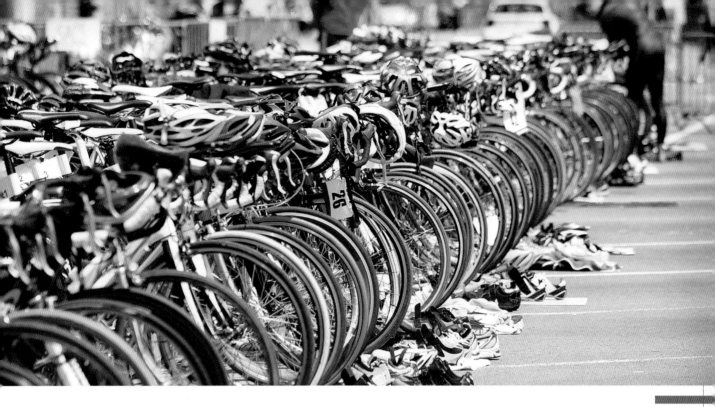

in fat and starches, and no new sauces, spices, or seasonings.

**Hydration:** Aim to take in half your body weight in ounces of fluid the day before your race. Try to drink throughout the day, evenly spreading out your fluid intake. For example, if you weigh 150 pounds (68 kg), try to take in 75 ounces (2.2 L), which can be broken down into drinking around 8 ounces (236.6 ml) of fluid every hour or 16 ounces (473.2 ml) every couple of hours. If it looks like it's going to be hot on race day and/or you are a heavy sweater, consider making that 75 ounces (2.2 L) a mix of water and sports drink, maybe 50 ounces (1.5 L) of water and 25 ounces (739.3 ml) of an electrolyte/carbohydrate solution. You can do more or less depending upon your specific needs, but don't go overboard with the water. Remember that your urine should be lightly colored, not necessarily clear.

## Race morning

Remember that eating breakfast is important to ensure that your fuel stores are adequately topped off before that starting gun goes off. Plan on eating roughly two hours or so before your race time to give your body time to digest and absorb the food.

As with your pre-race dinner, this meal should be very familiar to you. Ideally it will be a breakfast that you have tested time and time again in practice, before your longer brick workouts. Your body should be very accustomed to what you feed it so there are no surprises.

This meal can range from 200 to 500 calories of mainly carbohydrates, with a little protein as well to aid in the absorption. Two hundred calories is on the low end; most will probably need more. Don't overeat because you don't want to start the swim with an uncomfortably full stomach. If you have issues with stomach distress before workouts and find eating solid foods to be problematic, your breakfast can be in liquid form such as a shake or pre-made sports drink supplement.

You also don't want to overdo the hydration the morning of your race, either. There is nothing worse than feeling bloated as you stand waiting to start your triathlon. Consider drinking 10 to 16 ounces (295.7 to 473.2 ml) of fluid with your breakfast two hours or so before race start. This can be water or, if you feel you need additional calories and electrolytes and don't want to get them in solid food, choose a sports drink.

Then, ten to twenty minutes before the race start, drink another 8 to 10 ounces (236.6 to 295.7 ml) of water or sports drink. Some races will have water and even possibly sports drinks available in transition areas, but don't count on it, and plan on bringing it with you.

Eating your breakfast two hours or more before the race starts means you have gone a while without eating. Add in the thirty minutes or so that you are in the water, and the time starts to add up. If you feel like you will need a little more energy right before your Olympic tri, consider taking in another 100 to 200 calories ten to twenty minutes before the swim start. Once again, ideally these calories will come in liquid or semi-solid form, not solid food. The less work your

## FIVE PRE-RACE BREAKFAST EXAMPLES

1. **200 to 300 calories for a finicky stomach:** 150- to 200-calorie protein bar, 8 ounces (236.6 ml) water, and 8 ounces (236.6 ml) sports drink

2. **250 to 350 calories:** English muffin with 1 tablespoon (16 g) peanut butter, ½ cup (75 g) berries, 8 ounces (236.6 ml) water, and 8 ounces (236.6 ml) sports drink

3. **300 to 400 calories:** ½ cup (40 g) oatmeal (measured dry) with 1 tablespoon (20 g) honey, ½ cup (75 g) berries, 1 egg, 8 ounces (236.6 ml) water, and 8 ounces (236.6 ml) sports drink

4. **350 to 450 calories:** 6 ounces (170 g) low-fat Greek yogurt (if dairy pre-workout does not bother you) with ½ cup (40 g) granola, ½ cup (75 g) berries, 8 ounces (236.6 ml) water, and 8 ounces (236.6 ml) sports drink

5. **400 to 500 calories for a bigger appetite:** 1 whole wheat waffle toasted with 1 tablespoon (16 g) almond butter and 1 tablespoon (20 g) honey, 1 banana, 1 egg, 8 ounces (236.6 ml) water, and 8 ounces (236.6 ml) sports drink

body needs to do to digest this food before your race, the better. So ideally, these few hundred extra calories of energy might come from a sports drink, gel, or some other semi-solid nutrition product.

## T1

So you have finished your swim and are now getting ready to head out onto your almost 25-mile (40.2 km) bike ride. Now is a good time to get in some additional fluids to replace what you may have sweated out during the swim as well as to prepare you for the hour-plus bike ride. This is a good time to take a few seconds and swig 8 to 16 ounces (236.6 to 473.2 ml) of water or a sports drink so you don't have to worry about doing so at the start of the bike leg. The first few miles of the bike leg can be pretty congested as the race starts to spread itself out, so drinking while maneuvering through this traffic can be difficult. All too often, triathletes get caught up in the excitement of the race, failing to eat or drink anything until they are far into the bike course and have fallen behind nutritionally.

T1 can also be a great time to take in some energy, another 100 to 200 calories or so. I always recommend trying to keep these energy sources as easily digestible as possible, but you now have your choice of using a liquid form, solid energy bar, or similar food source. If you really want to eat something right after your swim, such as a few sport beans, blocks, or a half a bar, go for it. Your body is much better able to tolerate food while supported on a bike than while running on the ground. If you are someone who has difficulty drinking or eating while biking, doing so while in transition can be part of the solution for you. Front-load your nutrition if this works better for you.

## On the bike

Let's do some simple math. If you average 15 miles (24 km) per hour on the bike, your bike leg will take around 1 hour and 40 minutes to complete. Bike 20 miles (32.2 km) per hour, and you are done in roughly 75 minutes. I'll repeat this line over and over throughout the book because it is so important when it comes to racing triathlons. Repeat after me: The bike sets up the run.

The race doesn't end when you get off the bike. You have another 6.2 miles (10 km) to go. If you come off the bike under-fueled and dehydrated, this can and will dramatically affect the final leg of your race. Many people suffer during the run portion of their triathlons without realizing the primary cause is quite often poor nutrition, especially while on the bike.

So you need to take in calories and fluids during the bike leg, especially if you did not do so in T1. A rough estimate of caloric intake would be 250 to 400 per hour while on the bike. You can choose to bring these calories with you and/or supplement with what is given out at the aid stations along the bike course. I recommend being as self-contained as possible during your triathlons when it comes to your fueling, regardless of the distance. This doesn't mean that you can't and shouldn't make use of the aid stations, especially when it comes to hydration. You simply cannot always carry enough fluid with you. What it means is that relying on the aid stations to have exactly what you need, when you need it, can be a very risky bet: one you can't afford to lose.

That being said, I don't believe that "bonking" or running out of energy stores is a major concern when it comes to the sprint and Olympic distance triathlons. Unless you have severely restricted your caloric intake for days leading up to the race, your body should be able to perform without taking in significant extra calories during the race itself.

While the energy requirements of the two shorter distance triathlons are not as great as that of the half and full Ironman distance races, there is still the risk of dehydration and decreased performance. This is why consuming sports drink during the sprint and Olympic triathlons can be such a great strategy. The calories in the sports drink will provide extra energy and extra insurance against potential fueling issues, while hydrating at the same time.

So for a bike leg that takes a little over an hour, you might plan on taking in 300 extra calories. Twenty-four ounces (710 ml) of PowerBar Perform, a drink commonly found on race courses today, has 210 calories.

So if you had a gel in T1 containing 100 calories and drank one 24-ounce (710 ml) bottle of sports drink, you would have hit your 300 calorie total for the bike pretty easily.

And, since you want to hydrate with roughly 14 to 24 ounces (414 to 710 ml) of fluid per hour while on the bike, you would have also hit your fluid requirements if you fell somewhere in the middle of that range.

Carrying one 24-ounce (710 ml) water bottle filled with sports drink on your bike could satisfy both your fuel as well as hydration needs. That's pretty great.

Of course, there is a range depending upon your specific energy expenditure and sweat rate. I sweat like crazy, and my fuel requirements are higher than most.

## Basic bike fueling guidelines

**Fuel:** 250–400 calories per hour
**Fluid:** 14–24 ounces (414–710 ml) per hour

The primary goal of race-day nutrition for triathletes is to get off the bike having fueled and hydrated optimally. The bike is the "window of opportunity" you have to implement your plan and set yourself up to have the best run possible. You want to have taken in enough calories and nutrition to fuel your bike ride, while also leaving your fuel stores as full as possible to get you through the run.

You want to have to take in the least amount possible while running because the body is not a huge fan of eating and drinking while bouncing up and down for miles on end.

## T2

The range of finishing times for the 6.2-mile (10 km) run can be roughly forty to sixty minutes, so you still have a little work left to do. As in T1, T2 can be a great place to get in some quick calories, especially as your heart rate settles down a bit and makes it easier for your stomach to tolerate fuel.

That being said, if you fueled well during the bike ride, there is no reason to go crazy with your fueling while in T2. The faster a runner you are, the fewer calories you will most likely need at this point. If you think you will need extra calories before going out on the run, consider taking in a final 100 to 200 calories or so. Remember that your body doesn't like to have to digest food during running, so if you do take in calories, try to choose a semi-solid source such as a gel, sports beans, blocks, etc.

## The run

A good hydration strategy for the run leg of your Olympic tri is simply to take in fluids at the aid stations. Today, the vast majority of races have aid stations every 1 to 1½ miles (1.6 to 2.4 km) or so, perfectly spaced so you can take in fluids at regular intervals. Drinking 8 to 10 ounces (236.6 to 295.7 ml) or a cup's worth of fluid at every aid station is a good baseline strategy; if it is particularly hot, you may consider 1½ to 2 cups (236.6 to 473.2 ml).

Again, if you run a 7-minute mile (1.6 km), you are finished with the run in just over forty minutes. Average 10 minutes per mile (1.6 km), and your run will take a little more than an hour. Considering that most gels/block/sports beans and the like are to be consumed every thirty to forty-five minutes, you may want to take one in about halfway through your run, especially if you will be out there for forty-five minutes or more. The 100 calories or so along with the fluids you take in on the course can give you the final jolt you need to bring you all the way in.

## Basic run fueling guidelines

**Fluid:** 8 to 10 ounces (236.6 to 295.7 ml) of fluid every ten to twenty minutes
**Fuel:** 100 calories, ideally from a semi-solid source halfway through the run if necessary

## Post-race

You just put in a solid workout, exercising for two to three hours or more. If it's your first Olympic distance triathlon, that's a pretty big deal. I remember how I was a complete mess after my first Olympic distance tri for numerous reasons, including the fact that I did not refuel afterward. You want to enjoy your accomplishment as much as possible, and if you don't refuel afterward, I promise you that you won't feel your best. So take in some carbs, protein, and fluid as soon as you can, ideally within thirty to forty-five minutes, after crossing that finish line. Your body will thank you for it, and people you see soon afterward will say, "You did a tri? You don't look like you did anything at all!"

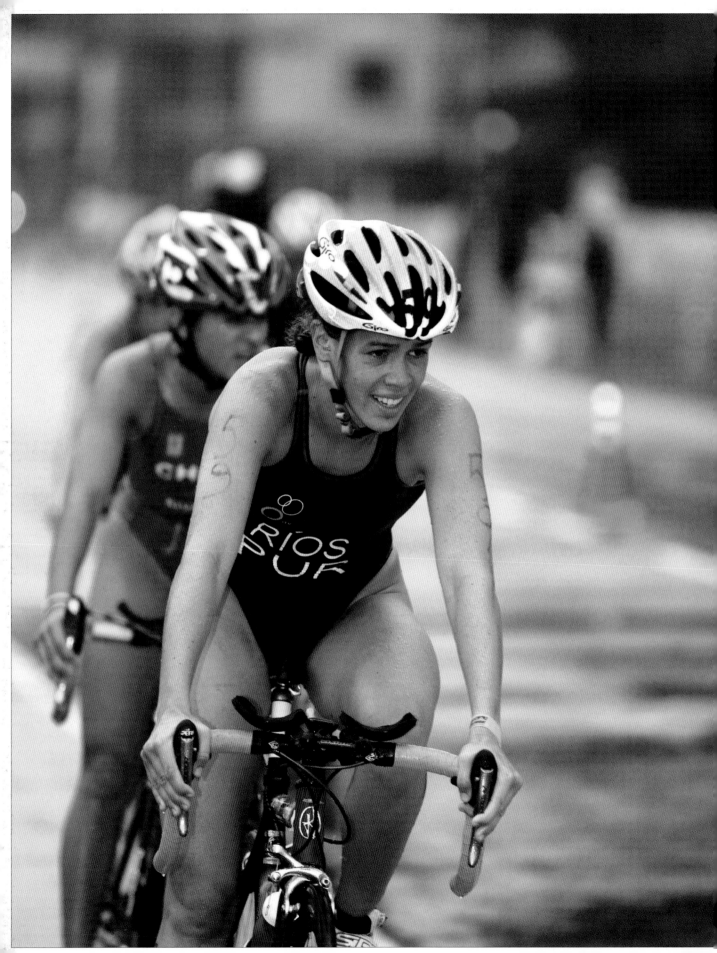

# Fueling Your Half-Iron Distance Triathlon

**SWIM 1.2 MILES (2 KM). BIKE 56 (90 KM).** Run a half marathon. The half Ironman distance triathlon is such a great challenge for most people, one that really starts to push the limits both mentally and physically. The pros and elites can now finish the half Ironman in around four hours, which is insanely fast, while the average person generally finishes in the neighborhood of five to six hours.

The swim might take somewhere around forty minutes, the bike three hours, and the run two hours, coming across the finish line in a little under six hours. That's a pretty long workout for the vast majority of people. To put it into perspective, according to marathonguide.com, in 2011, the average marathon finish times were four hours and twenty-six minutes for men and four hours and thirty-seven minutes for women. That means that, for many people, a half Ironman might take an hour longer to complete than a marathon (or even longer).

That's a pretty long time to ask our bodies to keep moving forward. Many triathletes want to hit a certain time goal as well. Therefore, if we worry about "hitting the wall" during a marathon, a race that generally takes less time to complete than a half Ironman, we better also take that into consideration when taking on a half Ironman triathlon.

The relative difficulty is what also makes the half Ironman such a great goal. It is hard, especially if you want to go as fast as you can. While some fit people can jump right into the sprint and Olympic triathlon distances and do relatively well on limited training, doing the same while going 70.3 total miles (113 km) can be much more difficult to achieve. It's hard to "fake" a half Ironman race performance. You need to devote time to some quality training, and you definitely need to have a solid nutrition strategy in place.

It's common sense: The longer your race distance, the greater your nutrition and hydration needs will be. You will be putting in some serious training in preparation for

2007 triathlon in Buenos Aires.

your half Ironman, burning a significant number of calories in training. If you don't pay attention to your pre-workout, workout, and post-workout strategies, it's not a question of if your performance will suffer on race day, just to what degree.

If you've read through the earlier chapters, you know this already. You've been eating healthier day to day while training. You've been fueling up for your workouts, dialing-in your race-day strategy during your longer brick workouts, and you've been sure to refuel after your workouts as well.

**IMPORTANT:**
"Practice doesn't make perfect. Perfect practice makes perfect."

This is such a powerful quote, and it holds true regardless of the sport. It's not enough to simply practice; you have to do what is known in sports psychology as "deliberate practice." Deliberate practice means that every workout has a specific goal and that you are training with purpose that will help you achieve success in your event. There is another simple way to put it: "You play like you practice."

Once again, far too many triathletes pay little to no attention to the fueling of their workouts, then wonder why they suffered or failed to hit their time goal during their triathlon. You cannot expect to implement something as important as fueling your body for an endurance event for the first time in the event itself without some major complications. Once you start stepping up to the half Ironman distance triathlon, dialing-in your race-day fueling strategy becomes that much more important. You want to have controlled as much as you could have during training, so your body is as accustomed as possible to the fueling plan on race day.

So if you are reading this book all the way through months before your event, which you should, realize that your race-day plan should be almost complete long before the race takes place. You will have experimented with your pre-workout meals, especially the meal before your long brick workout, and you will have figured out what works best for you and how long eating before the workout is optimal for your digestion. Maybe it's toast with peanut butter and a banana two hours before. Perhaps you prefer to stay liquid and have a specific carbohydrate drink or shake you consume three hours before. Whatever you have practiced with, that is what you will continue to take in on race day.

## Carbo-loading

Because they generally take one to three hours to finish, and energy depletion is not a huge concern, carbo-loading is not necessary for the sprint and Olympic distance triathlons. Going 70.3 miles (113 km) requires significantly more energy, however, and carbo-loading can provide the insurance you need to guarantee that your fuel stores are as full as possible. Remember that you should be tapering and doing significantly less exercise in the last few weeks leading up to your race, especially the last few days. If you are eating healthy and not burning as many calories through exercise, you are in essence increasing your carbohydrate stores without taking in any additional calories.

That being said, you should consider increasing your carbohydrate intake in the one to three days leading up to your half Ironman. This will help to top off your fuel stores and ensure that you have best prepared your body to go the distance.

You can do this two ways:

1. Eat additional carbs at each meal: You don't want to go crazy, but by consuming a little more carbohydrate at each of your five to six daily meals, you can get in the additional fuel without feeling bloated or overfed. One rule of thumb is to eat at the higher end of the daily range for carbs if you are not already, taking in around five grams per pound of half your body weight for the day.

   Carbohydrate-loading strategy: one to three days of half your bodyweight in pounds × five grams of carbs per day

   *Example:* 150-pound (68 kg) man: 75 pounds (34 kg) × 5 grams = 375 grams of carbs = 1,500 calories from carbs

2. Use a liquid supplement: In full disclosure, in my experimentation with carbohydrate-loading with well over one hundred long-distance triathlons and running events, I have found I prefer to carbohydrate-load with a liquid supplement drink. I eat my normal diet with perhaps a little extra carbs at each meal, but I also consume two or three store-bought carbohydrate drinks. They contain one hundred grams of carbs, some sodium, and nothing else. I definitely need to take in lots of extra carbs before my races, but I prefer to now get my additional carbs in liquid form to avoid the "heavy" feeling that eating these calories can create. I space them throughout the day, drinking one in the morning, one at lunch, and one in the evening. That's 300 grams of carbs and 1,200 calories in three quick bottles of liquid. If you are someone who cannot stomach carbing up with "real" food, you can consider using a liquid supplement to top off your tank. Be careful choosing a fruit-only drink because large amounts of fructose (fruit sugar) can cause some gastrointestinal distress if consumed in excess.

It bears repeating: If you plan on using something like these drinks as part of your carbohydrate-loading strategy, be absolutely sure to test it out on multiple occasions during your training. Plan on trying them out the day before your long brick or long run, drinking one to three, depending upon what you think you need, and see how your body reacts. Remember, trying this out on one occasion is not enough. Do this one-day liquid carbohydrate-loading test on at least three separate occasions, ideally many more.

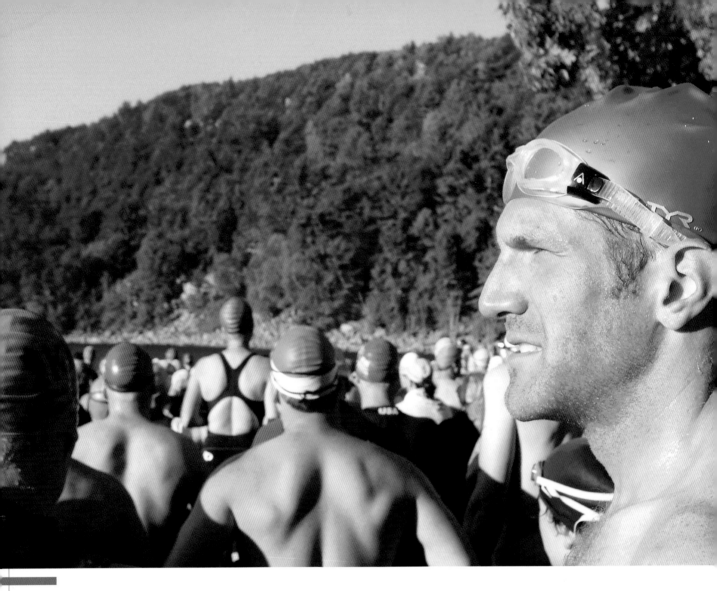

You want to focus on implementing, not inventing your fueling plan during your tri.

### Pre-race hydration

A familiar scene at endurance events is seeing triathletes walking around sipping endlessly from an ever-present water bottle in the days leading up to the race. You see this at the race expo, at the pre-race meeting, and at athlete registration. Soon you too might end up doing the same, thinking that if so many other people are doing it, I should be doing it, too.

Yes, you want to go into your race properly hydrated but, just like carbing-up before the race, there is no reason to overdo it. You are tapering, working out considerably less and therefore sweating less and losing less fluid in the last few days before your tri. Resist the urge to go crazy with your hydration, especially given the possibility of really overhydrating with water and running the risk of hyponatremia. I believe many carry the water bottle around and drink due more to the stress of the race than true hydration needs. The water bottle becomes their safety blanket.

Hydrate as you would normally do on any given day, taking in roughly half your body weight in ounces of fluid. You should drink throughout the day, but there is no reason to carry a water bottle everywhere you go.

## Pre-race sodium

As I discussed in the chapters on supplements and also hydration, it seems that sodium can play an important role in getting us to the finish line of our race. Once we start getting up to the half Ironman and Ironman distance triathlons, the role of sodium can become much more important.

Similar to taking in additional carbohydrates several days before the race to ensure we have optimally fueled up, consuming additional sodium is a similar technique used to combat the potential losses that can cause problems on race day. You might consider sodium-loading if the answer is yes to any or all of the following:

1. It will be extremely hot and/or humid during your tri.
2. You know that you are a salty sweater.
3. Your diet is particularly "clean" (i.e., you rarely eat processed foods and rarely add salt to your food).

If the answer was yes to any of the above, you may want to add a little extra sodium to your diet for one to three days before your race. Possible techniques are as follows:

1. Add a little extra salt to your food.
2. Snack on salty foods such as pretzels.
3. Take in a few salt tablets.
4. Make a sports drink part of your daily hydration plan.

## The day before

It's the day before your half Ironman, and you are probably going a little nuts from the taper. You are hydrating appropriately. You are adding some extra carbs into each meal, and perhaps you are even adding a little extra sodium to your daily diet. You are making sure to eat foods that are simple and that you are accustomed to eating. Excellent.

Nothing should change with your pre-race dinner. Keep it simple: Primarily carbs, try to eat on the early side, maybe 5 or 6 p.m. to give your body extra time to digest before your race, which often starts early in the morning.

## Race morning

One of the difficulties in taking in a pre-race breakfast is that the race time is often so early. Eating two hours before your official start time can be a challenge, especially for those people who have difficulty eating early. Add the pre-race jitters, and this can make taking in food that much more difficult.

It's a half Ironman, however, and you need to be properly fueled beforehand. If you ate dinner at 5 p.m. and woke up at 5 a.m. for a 7 a.m. race start, your body has been fasting for twelve hours. That's a long

1. 2 cups (280 g) pasta with marinara sauce, 4 ounces (113.4 g) grilled chicken, green beans (salted), 1 fruit, and water

2. Sandwich on whole wheat bagel with turkey, 2 percent cheese, veggies, and avocado or hummus, chicken noodle soup, 1 fruit, and water

3. Stir-fry with 2 cups (390 g) brown rice, some veggies (not a lot), 4 ounces (113.4 g) grilled chicken and soy sauce, 1 fruit, and water

If you do get hungry before bed or wake up in the middle of the night hungry, even after consuming your dinner, try to get in a snack that is dense with carbohydrate and sodium. The denser the food, the less you have to eat, thus avoiding the "heavy" feeling. So if you need a snack, try one of these quick, nutrient-rich snacks that only require a few bites:

1. A few peanut butter–filled pretzels

2. A handful of trail mix

3. A handful of granola with nuts

4. One-half of a higher-calorie energy bar containing carbs and protein

5. One to three peanut butter balls (Stir ½ cup [130 g] peanut butter and ⅓ cup [107 g] honey together. Then stir in 1 cup [80 g] oats and ½ cup [64 g] whey protein powder. Roll into twenty to twenty-four balls and refrigerate.)

time, and your liver glycogen stores are in fact depleted. Be sure to get in that pre-race breakfast you are accustomed to, eating it as soon as possible after waking up. That gives your body time to process it and gives you time to go to the bathroom beforehand as well.

Hydrate at this time as well, drinking 16 to 24 ounces (473.2 to 709.8 ml) of fluid along with your meal or shortly thereafter. If it's going to be a particularly hot day, you might also consider taking two salt tablets with this fluid as well.

## Before the race start

Bring an extra water bottle with you when you go to set up your transition. You can sip from this up until race time, or take in 8 to 10 ounces (236.6 to 295.7 ml) or more ten to thirty minutes before the start. If you are on the higher end of energy requirements and feel you need a little extra before you set out on your 70.3-mile (113 km) journey, consider taking in 100 quick calories or so from a semi-solid source such as an energy gel. If you want to avoid food as much as possible, sip sports drink while you set up your transition and drink 8 to 10 ounces (236.6 to 295.7 ml) or more ten to thirty minutes before your swim starts.

So now you are ready to race. You ate a good pre-race dinner the night before, consumed a quality breakfast, you hydrated as well, and maybe took in a little something extra like a quick gel before the gun goes off.

## T1

A 1.2-mile (2 km) swim is nothing to sneeze at for most people, and you still have 56 miles (90 km) left to bike and a half marathon to run as well. Faster swimmers will exit the water in thirty minutes or less; others will take around forty-five minutes or so to complete the swim.

T1 can be hectic, as people scramble like crazy to get on their bikes. It never ceases to amaze me how insane the transitions can be, especially in the longer distance triathlons such as the half and full Ironman distance races. Slow down and be smart while transitioning to the bike.

Taking in fluids or food right after a half Ironman swim can be problematic for some, easier for others. Some people come out of the water lightheaded and not wanting to eat or drink anything for a while. Others enter T1 and feel the need to take in something before they set out on the bike. Consider having an extra water bottle to grab a quick drink and possibly taking in a quick gel as well if you are someone who feels particularly depleted after swimming.

## The bike

The half Ironman distance is where the phrase "The bike sets up the run" is really significant. You are going to be on the bike for two to three hours or more and then need to run for several hours more after as well. That takes energy and a consistent fueling plan, which you have ideally practiced over and over in training. You should have a fueling and hydration schedule ready to go, and now it's just about making sure you implement it.

Many triathletes, myself included, need a little time for their stomachs to settle some after the swim before taking anything in.

I rarely consume anything in T1 and need to wait until I have been biking for five to ten minutes before starting to eat and drink. You don't want to wait too long, however, and fall behind in your nutrition strategy.

The general guidelines for fueling on the bike for your half Ironman are as follows.

## Basic bike fueling guidelines

**Fuel:** Thirty to sixty grams of carbohydrate (or more) per hour

**Fluid:** 14 to 24 ounces (414 to 709.8 ml) of fluid (or more) per hour

**Total calories:** 200 to 400 (or more) per hour

When it comes to utilizing the range of calories, this can be from a combination of total calories from sport drink, gels, liquid nutrition, and other sources.

**Example: Triathlete #1**

Goal: 300 calories per hour

Fluid: 20 ounces (591.5 ml) of fluid per hour Biking for 3 hours

20 ounces (591.5 ml) of a sports drink = 180 calories

One gel = 110 calories

So this person could kill two birds with one stone, combining her nutrition and hydration strategy, drinking one 20-ounce (591.5 ml) water bottle filled with sports drink and taking in one gel every hour for a total hourly caloric intake of 290 calories.

Here's a possible logistical strategy, assuming bike aid stations at mile 20 and mile 40:

- Start the bike with two water bottles filled with sports drink

- Carry one flask filled with three gels (in a jersey pocket or on the bike)

The triathlete would then finish both water bottles by mile 40, taking one additional bottle of sports drink from the final aid station. She is almost completely self-contained when starting the bike leg, carrying the bulk of both his nutrition and hydration with her.

I recommend trying to finish your nutrition and hydration with around ten minutes or so left on the bike. This will give your stomach time to settle before you make the transition to running, which the body isn't always happy about.

## Salt tablets

If you have determined you are a salty sweater and need to take in additional sodium in excess of what you will get in sports drinks, consider carrying tablets with you. A typical strategy would be to take one or two 250-milligram sodium tablets with fluid every hour or so while on the bike. If you feel muscle cramps coming on, take two more immediately.

## T2

There's nothing better than arriving at T2 during a triathlon, except of course crossing that finish line. The bike leg is where things can go wrong that could keep you from finishing the race, such as experiencing multiple flat tires and mechanical problems, so I am always relieved when I coast into T2 without any major issues.

You have biked more than 50 miles (80.5 km) and now have a pretty long run ahead of you, 13 miles (21 km), which can take anywhere from ninety minutes to two and a half hours or more. While your solid bike nutrition plan has set you up to have a great run, you still need to hydrate and take in some additional calories to get you through your half marathon.

I believe your caloric intake can be slightly less during the run leg of your half marathon than it was during the bike leg, for the following reasons:

1. You have consumed adequate calories while on the bike to fuel you for a portion of the run.

2. While 13 miles (21 km) is not a short distance, it is also not a full marathon. The average run time might be a little over two hours, which requires fueling but not marathon-level carbohydrate consumption.

3. The body generally tolerates taking in calories less well while running than it does while biking. You want to take in enough fuel, but you don't want to overdo it.

Just like in T1, you have the option of taking in fluid and fuel before you head out onto the run course. If you finished your fueling on the bike ten minutes or so before entering T2, this could be a good time to refuel. Consider having 10 ounces (295.7 ml) of water or sports drink and a gel or the equivalent. If it's a particularly hot day, you may want to take in a salt tablet or two.

## The run

One of your goals for your half Ironman distance race is to start your run feeling as good as possible. That may sound like common sense, right? Of course you want to feel good! Well, "good" doesn't necessarily mean you should feel like you just jumped out of bed. You have been racing for several hours and should be fatigued from the swim and bike legs. If you have paced the race correctly up until this point and fueled yourself well, you will still have the energy necessary to post a great bike split. If you pushed the bike too hard or under-fueled the race up until that point, you will definitely suffer on the run. If you did both, you could be in for a much slower finish time than you were shooting for.

What I love about the half Ironman distance tri is that it's just long enough to be really challenging, yet short enough that you can still race it pretty hard if you are so inclined. That can be a brutal combination, however, and makes fueling that much trickier as well as important.

Again, the faster you plan on running, the more likely you are to take in less fuel than someone running considerably slower. Your intensity will be higher, and you are also probably lighter and therefore have lower energy requirements. As with all general run guidelines, you want to take in fluid every ten to twenty minutes depending on the conditions and your needs. Most races will have the run aid stations spaced out at these intervals for you, generally every

1 to 2 miles (1.6 to 3.2 km). So you should aim on hydrating at all of them, taking in 10 ounces (295.7 ml) or more of fluid from sports drink and/or water.

You should also consider taking in additional calories to fuel your run from a more concentrated source such as a gel/block/sports bean–type source. Consuming 100 calories from one of these forms every thirty minutes or so can keep the glucose flowing to those working muscles and keep you from ending up shuffling across that finish line.

## SALT TABLETS

For half Ironman and Ironman distance races, I take salt tablets with me on both the bike and the run. If you are a big sweater and prone to cramping while running, I might consider increasing the frequency of your salt tablet intake, consuming one or two every thirty minutes or so and taking one or two if you feel cramps coming on at any time.

## Basic run fueling guidelines

**Fluid:** 8 to 10 ounces (236.6 ml to 295.7 ml) of fluid every ten to twenty minutes
**Fuel:** About 100 calories (twenty-five grams carb) ideally from semisolid source every thirty to forty-five minutes

## Post-race

Half Ironman triathlons require four to six hours or more of continuous hard exercise. Even while fueling yourself, you burn a significant number of calories and damage your muscles in the process. Refueling right after with carbs and protein will help to minimize the fatigue and feeling of being "beaten-up" afterward, expediting the recovery process and ensuring you will bounce back as quickly as possible. Ideally, try to get a carb-protein shake or snack within forty-five minutes after your race completion, but really, the sooner, the better. Then follow that up with a meal of carb and protein in the next two hours. I know that eating or drinking after a half Ironman can be the absolute last thing you want to do. I also know the feeling firsthand when you don't refuel and the feeling when you do. Trust me: The latter is exponentially better and well worth the few seconds it may take to guzzle down a recovery drink or suffer through a small meal.

You will take in the majority of your calories during the bike leg.

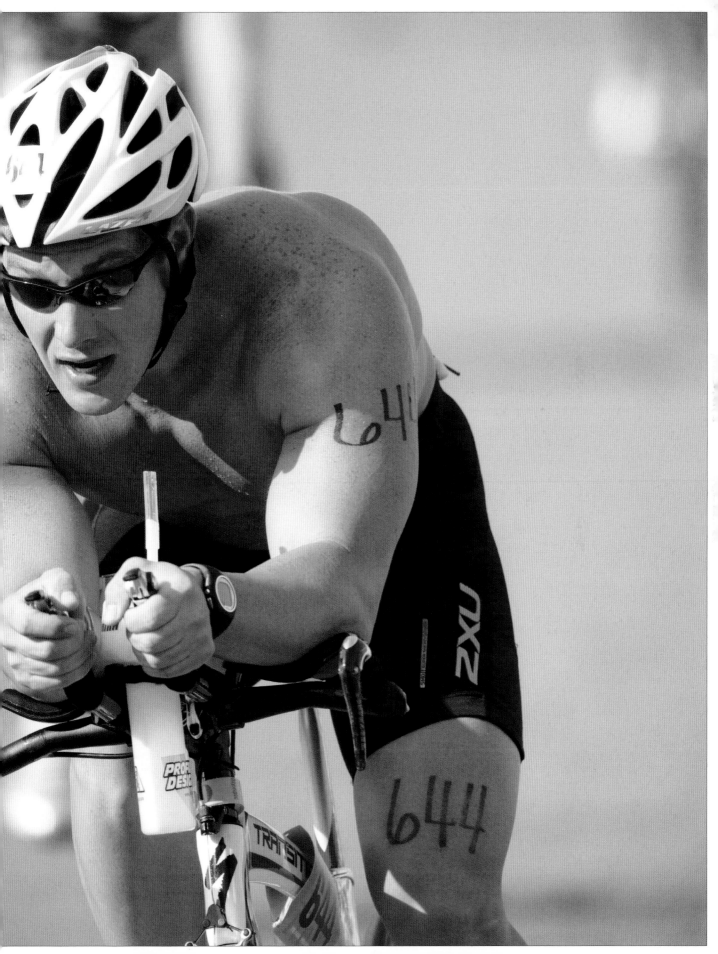

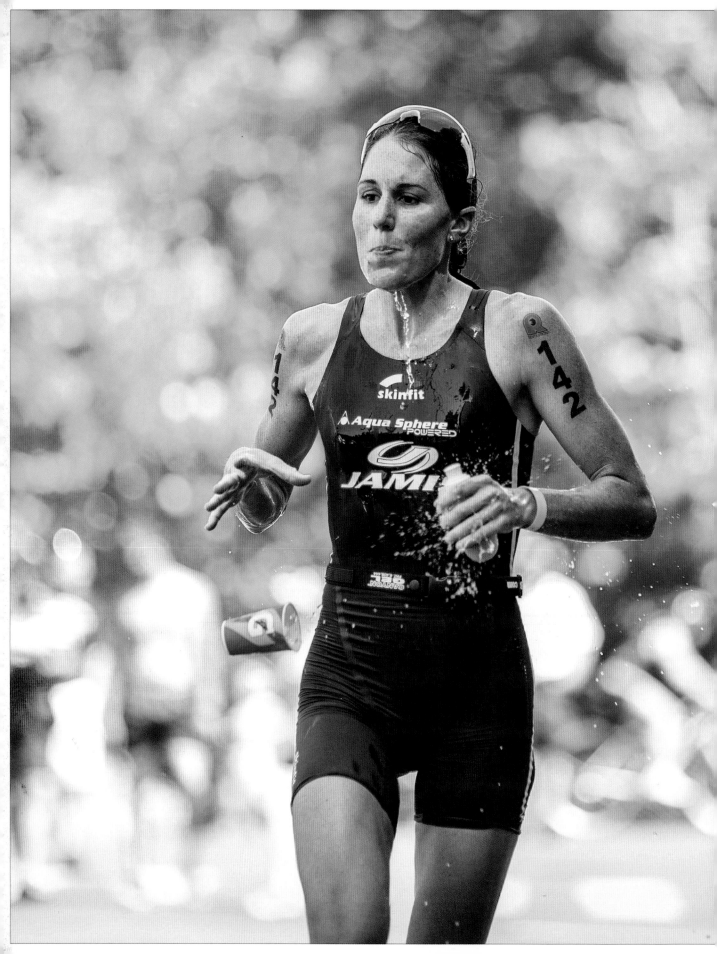

# Fueling Your Full-Iron Distance Triathlon

**I ABSOLUTELY LOVE THE IRONMAN** distance. For me, the shorter races are considerably more painful. Sprints are just way too short; I'm not even remotely close to being warmed up, and then the race is over. I have the same problem with the Olympic distance, and half Ironmans are still not the suffer-fest I truly enjoy, either. Ironman is the distance I personally love, the one with which I have the most experience, and the one I hope to do for many years to come.

While the shorter-distance triathlons are amazing events, and I have the utmost respect for those who excel at these distances, there is really nothing like the true endurance event. It challenges both the body and the mind. It rewards patience and planning and putting your ego aside. It's not about who goes the fastest; it's about who slows down the least. Going fast is often easy; not slowing down over long distances can be exponentially more difficult.

A huge part of what keeps us from slowing down is fueling.

An Ironman triathlete can burn approximately 8,000 calories or more on race day.

You "hit the wall" or slow down during an Ironman distance triathlon for three main reasons:

1. You didn't put in enough training.
2. You didn't pace yourself correctly.
3. You didn't fuel yourself correctly.

Many who race this distance make all three mistakes during their race, and then they continue to make them often over and over again. That's what makes racing 140.6 miles (226.3 km) such an incredible achievement; there is no perfect one-size-fits-all formula to any one of these variables. Training volume, how fast you push each of the three sports on race day, and what your fueling plan is—all of these are individualized concepts that must be experimented with and constantly refined over time.

Even pros such as Mark Allen and Chris McCormack struggled for years to put all three of these component parts together before they earned their Hawaii Ironman titles and began to dominate at the distance.

When it comes to the relative importance of these three concepts, improper fueling is usually to blame for the massive slowdown so many experience during an Ironman triathlon. They can't blame their training; there is no end of information on training plans, and most people generally get in the miles. Pacing can be more of an issue because many triathletes do go out too hard on the bike, but the long 112-mile (180.3 km) ride is a little too far for the average person to hammer through. No, the Bataan Death March that so many triathletes experience on the run courses of Ironman distance triathlons around the world is quite often the result of—you guessed it—improper fueling: not enough fuel, not the right fuel, not the right schedule of fuel, and yes, even too much fuel.

I can't stress enough how crucial it is for Ironman triathletes to properly fuel themselves during their event. No amount of mental toughness and no amount of training can override a body that is under-fueled and working on vapors. To bring back the simple car analogy; if you run out of fuel while driving a long distance, you slow down and eventually stop altogether. You wouldn't fill your gas tank up halfway before starting out on a long drive, and you definitely don't want to do so before trying to swim, bike, and run 140.6 miles (226.3 km).

Not only would you not set out on a long car ride without filling up your tank beforehand, but you would also have to make sure that you refilled along the way at periodic intervals. When the trip is long enough that a full gas tank simply won't be enough to get you all the way to your final destination, refueling along the way is not an option but a necessity. This simple analogy is exactly how you need to approach your Ironman distance triathlon fueling strategy. You cannot afford to start the journey under-fueled, and you have to refuel along the way. Fail to do either one, and your trip won't be a very pleasant one.

When it comes to fueling the shorter-distance triathlons, the fueling plan is more about maximizing your potential. Fueling up beforehand and even during is not ultimately focused on getting you to the finish line as much as it is allowing you to have your best race possible. In other words, you can make small mistakes with your plan at these distances and while your performance will suffer, the repercussions are relatively small. It's tough to under-fuel your sprint distance triathlon. While race hydration is always something you should pay attention to, it's not half as important during your Olympic distance race as it is your Ironman distance. In other words, when your goal is to fuel a 140.6-mile (226.3 km) journey, every single aspect of your fueling plan is essential to your success. Carbohydrate-loading, pre-race dinner, pre-race breakfast, and your race nutrition—every one of these elements needs to be focused on, and their correct implementation will determine whether or not you suffer or excel on race day. The choice is yours.

## Carbohydrate-loading

If there is ever a time to load up on carbs, it's before an Ironman triathlon. The race will take most people anywhere from ten to seventeen hours to complete, and that takes a significant amount of energy. Since the body can only store roughly 2,000 calories in the form of glycogen (stored carbohydrate), and an Ironman triathlete can burn 7,000 calories or more during the course of the event, that's pretty simple math. You need to make sure you enter the water with your tank full, and you darn well better take in a boatload of calories along the way as well.

A huge part of properly fueling your body for the Ironman distance is carbohydrate-loading. This entails taking in extra calories in the form of carbohydrates in the final few days leading up to your race. If you are tapering correctly and eating well to begin with, you are already carb-loading to an extent because you are not burning as many calories due to your dramatically decreased training volume. While some think that the taper effect is enough to fully load your fuel stores, I do not. Of course, much of this has to do with how much carbohydrate your normal diet consists of, but for the vast majority of people, taking in additional carbohydrates right before their Ironman triathlon is essential.

My best races came after I began dialing-in my carbohydrate-loading strategy. Although it wasn't a triathlon, I had my first real breakthrough race when I did the "Run to the Sun" ultra-marathon on Maui, a 36-mile (58 km) run from sea level to the 10,000-foot (3,048 m) summit of the volcano Mt. Haleakala. I was experimenting with a new three-day liquid carbo-loading strategy, eating my normal meals while supplementing with this new drink. It worked incredibly well, and while I obviously took in fuel on the race course, I knew I had fueled up pre-race better than I ever had before.

You need to make sure your body has the optimal amount of fuel in the form of glycogen in your liver and muscle "tanks" when you arrive on that starting line. In the final three days leading up to your race, you should consider adding extra carbs to each meal, by either increasing portion sizes, taking in additional forms of carbs, or both. I tend to do both. My pasta portions are slightly larger, and I also supplement throughout the day with a few special carbohydrate drinks.

### CARBOHYDRATE-LOADING PLAN

- Start increasing your carbohydrate intake in the last one to three days leading up to your race.
- Consider supplementing with additional forms of carbohydrate, ideally liquid or semisolid forms.
- Consume anywhere from 400 to 1,000 additional calories or more above your normal daily intake.
- Consume simple foods that you are accustomed to eating—nothing new.

If you are thinking of supplementing with a store-bought carbohydrate product, be sure to try it out in training on multiple occasions. For example, if you have a long brick on a Saturday, test it out with a day of carbo-loading on Friday. Do this before as many of your long brick workouts and long runs as possible. You want to know far ahead of time that these forms of carbohydrates work for you.

## Pre-race sodium-loading

Does lack of sodium cause muscular cramping? If we take in extra sodium, can our bodies "store" it for our race like it does carbohydrates? The answer to both questions is maybe. There still is a debate concerning both issues. You can find experts who will argue back and forth about whether or not the lack of sodium is one of the causes of those horrible cramps, as well as whether or not taking in extra sodium before we exercise is a worthwhile endeavor.

It's been my experience that sodium does make a big difference during endurance events, for both myself and my clients. Numerous sports nutrition companies, who spend large amounts of money conducting research on sports performance, are adding extra sodium to many of their products. And the vast majority of professional triathletes, the ones whose livelihoods depend on them performing their very best, have sodium supplementation as part of their race nutrition plan.

Many triathletes, myself included, also eat fairly "clean" the majority of the time,

avoiding processed foods that are jam-packed with sodium, and rarely, if ever, add salt to their foods. Add being a "salty sweater" to the mix, and my sodium levels might be lower than most. If your race is going to be particularly hot and/or humid, you might consider adding a little extra salt to your diet in the final few days leading up to your Ironman triathlon.

## Techniques for sodium-loading

1. Snack on salty foods such as pretzels.
2. Hydrate with sports drinks.
3. Supplement with salt tablets.

Don't overdo it. You will still be taking in sodium on race day. Just add a little more to your diet for a few days.

## Pre-race hydration

If there's one message that seems to have gotten through when it comes to endurance events, it is the practice of hydrating before a race—even more so than hydrating during the race. It's probably because it's much easier to sit around and drink a Gatorade in front of the TV or in your car than it is while at mile 78 of your Ironman bike leg in 90-degree (32.2° C) heat. Water bottles become like pacifiers for a baby in the mouths of triathletes and most likely for the very same reason: the calming effect more so than the hydration.

While you should hydrate before your race, there is no need to take in more than your normal hydration needs. Remember the urine test: Your pee should look like lemonade, not much darker and yet not clear, either. You should not feel like you are taking in considerably more fluids than you normally do in these last few days. Spread out your fluid intake throughout the day and consider mixing it up—some sports drink and some water.

## Hydration guidelines

- Half your body weight in ounces of fluid
- Consider taking in water and sports drink

## Bike/gear check-in

Ironman distance races require more pre-race athlete preparation given their extreme race distance. Part of this preparation includes "checking" certain things in the day before the race. Now, each race is different in the way in which they do things, so be sure to read the *Athlete's Guide* cover-to-cover and attend the race meeting if they have one. Failure to do either one of these things can leave you open to a potential nightmare come race time due to your failure to follow proper procedures.

I have to admit that the twenty-plus Ironman distance races I have done to date have all been Ironman-branded events. Ironman has a certain way of doing things, and I'd argue they put on a great race. There are now numerous Ironman distance races put on by different race companies, but I will use the way the World Triathlon Corporation, the company that puts on Ironman-branded events, structure their races to give you a basic idea of how things are most often structured.

You will most likely receive several bags at registration, quite often five different bags, each with a definitive purpose. At Ironman, they usually are as follows:

1. **Dry Clothes bag:** This bag is what I use to bring all my race-day nutrition down to transition the morning of the race. This includes a sports drink to sip on before the swim and my bike bottles filled with my carb fuel that will go on the bike. You will also use this bag to put on whatever you are wearing down to the swim start such as sweatpants, sweatshirt, flip-flops, or a warm hat—whatever you bring down to transition that you won't need once the race starts. There is often a place to drop the bag off right near the swim start, and you will get this bag back after you cross the finish line.

2. **Swim-to-Bike bag:** This is the bag you will get in T1 and will hold everything you need for your bike ride. It will also hold any food or drink that you want to take in T1 before you go out on your 112-mile (180.3 km) bike ride. As far as nutrition goes for the bike ride itself, the majority of my nutrition is already on the bike in bike bottles. In addition, I often put a flask filled with several gels and a tube filled with salt tablets in this bag. I put both in the pockets of the tri top that I wear under my wetsuit during the swim and then wear on the bike as well.

3. **Bike-to-Run bag:** Everything you need for the run, you will put in this bag along with whatever nutrition you want to take in while in T2. Gear may include your

sneakers, a hat/visor, a Fuel Belt if you use one, clothes if you plan to change, etc. Given the vast offerings at the aid stations of most Ironman races, I have simplified what I bring along with me during the run as far as nutrition. I used a Fuel Belt myself for many of my earlier Ironman races; now I just bring another gel flask and another tube of salt tablets with me. I carry the flask in one hand and put the salt tablets in my tri top pocket.

4. **Special Needs bike:** Some races allow you to pack a bag with additional nutrition that will be available for you to pick up roughly halfway through the bike ride. While I personally do not use the special needs bags, many triathletes do. These bags can hold whatever you would like: additional gels, powders, bars, whatever you may want around mile 56. You can also use these bags as insurance, putting in extra nutrition in case a valuable water bottle full of nutrition gets launched during your ride, you spill your salt tablets, or something else unexpected occurs.

5. **Special Needs run:** Similar to the special needs bag for the bike, you can pack this bag with whatever nutrition you may want at the half-marathon point of your run. Additional gels, sports beans, blocks, bars, an energy drink—whatever you have used in training that you don't want to carry with you but might want halfway through the final leg of your Ironman distance race.

Once again, not all races offer these bags, but many do. You usually drop your bike off the day before the race in transition along with your Swim-to-Bike and Bike-to-Run bags. Then, the morning of the race, you bring your Dry Clothes bag to the start along with your Special Needs Bags if you plan to use them.

When I first started doing Ironman races, you were not allowed to access your Swim-to-Bike or Bike-to-Run bags on the morning of the race. This meant that whatever nutrition you planned on putting in these bags had to be put in the night before. This occasionally proved to be problematic, especially if you forgot to put some essential item in or if these bags lay out in the sun and heat for a day, "baking" all your nutrition in the process.

Things have changed for the better, however, since I did my first Ironman race well over a decade ago. Even though most races still have you drop off your Bike and Run bags the day before, you are now able to access them the morning of the race. This is a huge deal. So you can bring your gels, bars, and so on down the morning of the race and put them in these bags without worrying about forgetting them the night before or having them sit out in the elements for too long.

## Pre-race dinner

Many Ironman races have "Athlete Dinners," pasta parties either one or two nights before the event, especially at the destination races. These meals usually consist of simple foods such as salad, bread, and pastas with plain sauces. Race directors realize that the athletes know they shouldn't eat anything

## DESTINATION RACES—BRING FOOD WITH YOU

I have participated in Ironman races around the world. When traveling to a foreign country, finding foods that are familiar can be extremely difficult, and if you will be traveling for your Ironman, you need to plan accordingly. This goes for your entire race nutrition plan: what you will eat in the days leading up to the race, your pre-race breakfast, race nutrition, everything.

When my race involves plane travel, I now pack a box and ship my nutrition to the race site ahead of time. To do this is relatively inexpensive, even to countries as far away as New Zealand and South Korea. It ensures I have everything I need, both food for the days prior, such as oatmeal, energy bars, and powdered drink mixes, as well as my race-day nutrition.

It also alleviates the incredible hassle and potential costs associated with trying to bring nutrition with you on the plane and then drag it halfway around the world. Pack up as much as you can, wrap it with as much bubble wrap as you can, and send it on its way. I have done this well over a dozen times with no problems whatsoever except for Ironman China. The box I sent to my hotel on Hainan Island was held up upon arrival in China due to it being a "suspicious package" and was never released to me but arrived back home at my doorstep several months later. That taught me the lesson of shipping the bulk of my nutrition ahead of time but also carrying a few absolutely essential nutrition products with me.

too different before their triathlon, and therefore, the dinner fare is relatively simple.

I have attended many of these pre–Ironman dinners over the years, especially overseas. These get-togethers are often scheduled two days before the race because the race directors realize that most of the athletes want to eat their own pre-race dinners and get to bed on the early side. They are often more than just a dinner, with different speakers, videos, and the like. They can be a great way to get in the spirit of the race and meet fellow triathletes.

That being said, if your Ironman race has a dinner and you do attend, be sure to only eat foods that you are accustomed to. Do not try anything new and stick with foods you are the most familiar with eating. Don't pig out, either!

The night before the race, you should eat a medium-size dinner: some form of carbohydrates with a little bit of protein. You will most likely be going to bed earlier than normal, so eat earlier as well. This will also allow your body extra time to digest the meal before your race start. Stay away from fats and starches, foods that are more difficult to digest.

So you have had a good simple dinner, and you went to bed early but probably tossed and turned all night in restless anticipation of tomorrow's big event. You also most likely set your alarm clock for a wake-up time that used to be when you were coming home from a late party, not getting up to go push your body for 140.6 (226.3 km) miles.

You will ideally get up two hours or more before your race start. Even though you might not be hungry in the least, try to eat immediately after waking up. This will give your body time to digest as much as possible and give you time to go to the bathroom, most likely several times or more. Eat and then start getting everything together to get down to your race site.

## THREE HOURS?

Some coaches recommend getting up at least three hours before your race. I think that this is unnecessary for many, and I don't like to do it, either. If you feel like you do need a little extra time to process your food but also want to get as much sleep as possible, consider doing what I do. I leave one of my 400-calorie/100-gram carbs store-bought drinks by my bed before I turn in. I inevitably toss and turn and wake up sometime in the middle of the night, so I just roll over, chug down the contents of the bottle, and then go back to sleep.

## Pre-race breakfast

It's race morning. Your alarm clock woke you, and you popped out of bed, probably more than a little stressed at how little sleep you got the night before. No worries; one rarely sleeps the night before an Ironman. It's the sleep two nights before that really matters, anyway.

Now is the time to get in your pre-race breakfast, the final meal before you set out on your 140.6-mile (226.3 km) journey, a meal that you have used time and time again and that your body knows well. Eat it as soon as you can so you can focus on all the other tasks at hand. Don't worry if you feel a little (or a lot) nauseated because this

is often due to pre-race jitters. Force yourself to eat that breakfast. In about six hours, you'll be really glad you did.

Once again, this breakfast should consist almost entirely of carbohydrates, have minimal protein and fats, and be somewhere around 400 calories, more or less depending upon your needs and what you have practiced with in training before your long workouts.

It's a good idea to hydrate with breakfast. Once again, do not overdo it. Take in somewhere between 16 to 24 ounces (473.2 to 709.8 ml) of fluid, especially if it's going to be a particularly hot day.

## FIVE PRE-IRONMAN BREAKFAST EXAMPLES

1. Large bagel with 1 to 2 tablespoons (16 to 32 g) peanut butter (add honey if you need more carbs), one banana, 8 to 16 ounces (236.6 to 473.2 ml) water, and 8 ounces (236.6 ml) sports drink

2. ½ cup (40 g) oatmeal (measured dry) with ¼ cup (38 g) berries, 1 tablespoon (20 g) honey, 1 tablespoon (9 g) chopped nuts, one egg, 8 to 16 ounces (236.6 to 473.2 ml) water, and 8 ounces (236.6 ml) sports drink

3. 1 whole wheat waffle toasted with 1 tablespoon (16 g) almond butter and 1 tablespoon (20 g) honey or syrup, fruit smoothie with one-quarter scoop whey protein powder, 1 cup (155 g) fruit, 4 ounces (118.3 ml) juice and water/ice to liking, 8 ounces (236.6 ml) water, and 8 ounces (236.6 ml) sports drink

4. Ready-to-drink lactose-free shake (200 to 300 calories) with carbohydrate and protein, one banana, (add a granola bar if you need more calories), and 8 ounces (236.6 ml) sports drink

5. Finicky stomach: 200- to 300-calorie protein bar, one banana, and 16 to 24 ounces (473.2 to 709.8 ml) sports drink (if you need more calories, add something simple such as a granola bar or dry cereal)

## Caffeine: Can I have my Joe?

I have very few vices left in this world; caffeine is one of them. As I discussed in the chapter on supplements, caffeine is indeed an "ergogenic aid," a performance enhancer in numerous ways. Some professional triathletes opt to go off caffeine several weeks before their race for two reasons: One, it allows them to monitor their body more closely during the final lead up to the race, resting when need be and not having the false sense of energy that caffeine can provide. Second, by weaning themselves off the stimulant for a few weeks, it is believed to increase the ergogenic effects on race day, providing a much more potent boost than if it had been used all the way through training.

I understand the reasons for choosing to eschew caffeine before an Ironman. They are both solid arguments. But in my case, it's just not happening. I'm not giving up my morning pot of coffee, especially during the taper phase when life is hard enough due to the massively decreased training volume and subsequent bad moods and crankiness. That being said, if you are tougher than I am and want that added edge during your Ironman, consider cutting out the caffeine a few weeks before race day. That way when you do take it in, possibly in your gels and by consuming soda offered on the run course, it may have an increased positive effect on your race, especially when it matters most.

## Before the race starts

Okay. So now you have carbo-loaded for several days. You stuck to your daily hydration plan, you added a little extra sodium to your diet, you had a pre-race dinner and a pre-race breakfast that were extremely familiar to you and primarily carbohydrates, and you drank a little fluid before you set out for the race start.

Your fuel stores should be topped off. You are good to go.

As you make your way to the transition and body-marking area, you may want to bring one final drink and possibly some form of carbohydrate snack for right before the race. You can take in 8 to 10 ounces (236.6 to 295.7 ml) or so of water or sports drink ten to thirty minutes before the swim start, and you may even feel you need one final 100-calorie "hit" of a gel or other semi-solid product ten to thirty minutes before the race start as well. Just remember that the closer you get to the start of the race, the less solid you want your form of nutrition to be.

## T1

There is nothing better than exiting the swim of an Ironman, especially for guys like me for whom the swim is their least favorite discipline by far. Depending on how good a swimmer you are, you could have been in the water for anywhere from one to two hours, and when you exit the swim, it can take a little while to get your land legs back. Know that, if you want, T1 is a time to take in some fluids and calories if you wish to before you get on the bike. For me, I am too

### WHEN IN DOUBT, PUT IT IN

If you think you might want some nutrition in T1, but you're not quite sure, put it in your bag. If you want it, it's there. If you don't feel like consuming anything after the swim, then just leave it in your bag. It is much better to have it and leave it than to want it and not have it. It's a long day, and you want as many options as possible.

disoriented after the swim to want to take in anything at all in the first transition, but that doesn't mean you shouldn't. You have a 112-mile (180.3 km) bike ride ahead of you, and if you want to take some nutrition in before setting out on your five-hour-plus bike leg, then by all means take a few extra seconds in T1 and take it in. If you plan on doing so, this would be nutrition that you had put in your Swim-to-Bike bag earlier that morning.

## The bike

The first few miles of the Ironman bike can be a little stressful. You just exited a 2.4-mile (4 km) swim, rushed through transition with hundreds of other triathletes, and are now out on the bike course with a long day ahead of you. Your heart rate is most likely elevated, and your adrenaline is pumping. It can be a good idea to wait a few miles before you start to implement your nutrition plan, giving your body time to settle down.

If you have trained correctly, your nutrition plan on the bike should be automatic by race day. You practiced it during your long bike rides and your brick workouts, refining it over the past few months, and now all that hard work is about to pay off.

You should be taking in calories and fluids on a set schedule. Small sips of fluid are better than big gulps. You have a pretty long bike ride ahead of you, so spreading food and fluid intake over the next five to seven hours or more shouldn't be too difficult. Hydrating and taking in calories every ten to fifteen minutes can be a good "feeding" schedule for many triathletes.

Here's an example of a bike nutrition plan I used for one of my last Ironman races: On the bike, I brought the following:

- One bike bottle filled with 1,200 liquid calories
- One bike bottle filled with 125 calories of sports drink
- One gel flask filled with 400 calories

So I had a total of 1,750 calories. My goal was to bike a 5:15 bike split, so I had around 330 calories per hour "on board" with me starting out.

I have found I usually need 400 calories or more per hour while on the bike, so I was still a little short. I planned on killing two birds with one stone, taking in additional calories while hydrating with a sports drink from each aid station. The aid stations were roughly 20 miles (32.2 km) apart. I was shooting to hit these stations in a little less than an hour, and each bottle of sports

drink from the aid station would be another 125 calories or so.

So I would grab four additional bottles of sports drink along the way, at miles 20, 40, 60, and 80. I had found through racing experience that I get a little bloated by the end of the ride, so I planned on switching to water at mile 100 for the last aid station to allow my stomach to settle down for the run. So four bottles of sports drink at roughly 125 calories each would come out to an additional 500 calories.

**1,750 calories on the bike + 500 calories from the aid stations = 2,250 calories**

**2,250 calories ÷ 5.25 hours biking = 430 calories per hour**

My plan is usually to take something in every ten minutes while on the bike, alternating between taking in fluid and taking in calories. I would also take in one gel and two salt tablets every hour on the bike. Biking at a little over 20 miles (32.2 km) per hour would get me to the aid stations roughly every hour, so I would use them as a reminder to consume the gel and salt tablets. So here's how an hour on the bike might look:

**Ten minutes:** two swigs of sports drink
**Twenty minutes:** one swig of liquid calories
**Thirty minutes:** two swigs of sports drink
**Forty minutes:** one swig of liquid calories
**Fifty minutes:** two swigs of sports drink
**One hour:** [first aid station]

- Toss empty sports drink bottle and take a new one.
- Take in one gel from gel flask.
- Take two salt tablets.

I would basically repeat this schedule for the entire bike ride. I would only deviate from it for three reasons: One, if later in the bike ride, the sports drink started to become difficult to get down; I would then switch to water until my stomach settled down. Two, if I started to feel any signs of a cramp coming on, I would take additional salt tablets immediately. Three, even though it may seem on the higher end of calories per hour, I have occasionally found myself needing even more energy and taking a few extra gels at the later aid stations.

That is my plan: Yours will be different. The key point here is that it is just that, a *plan*—a schedule that you have practiced in training and that you will implement like clockwork on race day. Here are the basic ranges for fueling your Ironman distance bike ride:

**Fuel:** 250 to 400 or more calories per hour

**Fluid:** 14 to 24 ounces (414 to 709.8 ml) of fluid (or more) per hour

How much you take in each hour depends on a variety of factors, including your weight, pacing, tolerance, and more. My philosophy is that, if you are going to make a mistake, especially during an Ironman distance triathlon when fueling is crucial, err on the side of too much rather than too little, especially if you are a first-timer. Being over-fueled means potential stomach aches and gastrointestinal distress, two conditions that are uncomfortable but that you can push through, and they can pass.

If you run out of fuel and "bonk," however, or become dehydrated, the consequences are much more severe. Better to feel a little full at mile 90 on the bike and back off your feeding plan rather than burn through your fuel reserves and limp into T2, only to have a full marathon left ahead of you.

Your goal should be to finish taking in your calories with a few miles or more left on the bike leg. This will give your stomach time to process what is left before you ditch the bike and have to finish the race on foot.

Let me say it one last time because it is so darn important: **The bike sets up the run**.

The success of your nutrition plan while on the bike is one of the defining factors in how your overall race will play out. Do a great job of fueling while biking, and your run will be exponentially easier. Fail to adequately take in the necessary calories, fluids, and electrolytes, and your run will most likely be turned into the "Ironman shuffle."

## T2

You just basically spent half a day eating and biking over the course of 112 miles (179.2 km), so chances are you're not going to be ravenous when you enter T2. It's usually just the opposite. That being said, if you think you want some additional special type of fuel after the bike, put it in your bag so you have it available to you when you enter T2. As I said earlier, I have another gel flask and tube of salt tablets in my bag. That's the extent of the additional nutrition I bring with me on the run.

You may use a Fuel Belt for the run as I did for my first few Ironman races to carry fluids, additional calories, salt tablets, and so on. Most of these items will often be available to you on the course, but if

## GASTROINTESTINAL DISCOMFORT

Let's face it: Doing an Ironman distance triathlon is difficult for everybody. I believe it's almost equally as difficult for the winner as it is for the last person to officially run across the finish line.

One part of what makes it so hard is the distance you must travel to finish; the second part is how difficult it can be to fuel yourself along the way. I believe that because it can be difficult to fuel yourself over 140.6 miles (226.3 km), you have to expect a certain amount of gastrointestinal distress along the way. It comes with the territory. For me, it generally comes around mile 80 of the bike, when I often start to essentially throw up the sports drink when I try to get it down and have to switch over to water. I know I needed to take in that much up to that point, I know that I will still need to drink throughout the race, and I also know that the discomfort is just part of the whole tough journey that is the Ironman triathlon. My point is that even if you are fueling yourself correctly, almost *if* you are fueling yourself correctly, you will most likely feel gastrointestinal distress at some point during the race. Just like a cramp or a nagging pain, you put it out of your mind and you keep moving forward.

you have used it in training and prefer a specific type of nutrition that will not be offered, then by all means wear one for the run. I think this is actually a good idea for first-time Ironman triathletes who often use these belts while in training.

As I said earlier, one of my early strategies was to use a four-bottle belt, each bottle holding two gels pre-mixed with fluid. That made it easy for me to take in the gels at my own pre-set intervals anywhere on the course, without having to wait and take it with fluid at an aid station.

Quite often, your race may have fluids right there in T2 for you to grab on the way out if you so desire. If you feel like you need something before you hit the first aid station, take a few extra seconds in T2 and grab a cup or two of fluids. This can also be a good time to take a salt tablet or two, especially if it's turning out to be a particularly hot day.

## The run

The infamous Ironman run—when you're feeling good, it's one of the greatest experiences in the world. When you're feeling horrible, it's like a long, slow death march. I like to think of the marathon as just one-mile runs, from aid station to aid station.

The logistics of fueling during an Ironman triathlon run has become significantly easier over the years thanks to great organizations such as the World Triathlon Corporation that put on the races. They have taken all the worry and hassle of having to carry all your nutrition with you, so you can just run.

Many of the races have the aid stations spaced out every 1.5 miles (2.4 km) or so, perfect intervals to take in fluids along the way. They also offer numerous different types of carbohydrate-based foods for you to fuel up with at periodic intervals as well.

Here is what was offered at the aid stations on 2013 Ironman Lake Placid run course, approximately every mile (1.6 km):

Powerbar Perform

Water

Bananas

Bonk Breaker Bars

GU Original Energy Gels

Roctane Ultra Endurance Gels

GU Chomps

Chicken broth (after dark)

Pretzels

Fruit

Cola

A simple fueling strategy during the run would be as follows, assuming aid stations every 1.5 miles (2.4 km) along the course:

- Drink 1 to 2 cups (236.6 to 473.2 ml) of fluid every aid station. Choose sports drink over water if possible until your stomach tells you otherwise.
- Take in 100 calories from an energy gel, block, sports beans, or the like every thirty to forty-five minutes.
- Take one or two salt tablets every thirty to sixty minutes, depending upon the conditions and your needs.
- If you feel cramps coming on, take one or two salt tablets immediately.

Cola: As I talked about earlier, caffeine is a performance enhancer and a potentially powerful one at that, especially during the final leg of an Ironman triathlon. The strategy of many is to hold off drinking the "defizzed" soda until you absolutely need it, when you really start suffering during the run. The effects of caffeine at this point can be nothing short of amazing, mentally as well as physically. The other rule, however, is that once you start drinking it during the run, you need to continue to do so for the remainder of the race or risk the caffeine crash that can come from stopping. I tend to start drinking cola around the halfway point of the marathon; it's a great thing to look forward to and can be a "secret weapon" when you need it most.

If you don't drink caffeine regularly, however, it's probably not a great idea to start during an Ironman triathlon.

## Post-race

One of the last things most people want to do after finishing their Ironman triathlon is eat or drink anything. The mere sight of a sports drink or energy bar can make you want to throw up. You just burned an insane amount of calories, however, and the rules of refueling still apply, if not significantly more so after your Ironman.

Many races have a food tent at the finish where you can refuel immediately after completing your race. If you can stomach it, it will help your recovery to refuel with the same types of foods and fluids that you would after a long workout. I like to bring a recovery drink to the start with me and put it in my Dry Clothes bag so I can have it right after I finish. You should also try to replace fluids with a bottle or two of water or sports drink after as well. If you plan on drinking alcoholic beverages to celebrate your incredible achievement, definitely try to refuel first. If you refuel and rehydrate after your Ironman, you will help expedite the recovery process and feel much better when you wake up the following morning. You'll still feel like you've been beaten up, just not quite as badly.

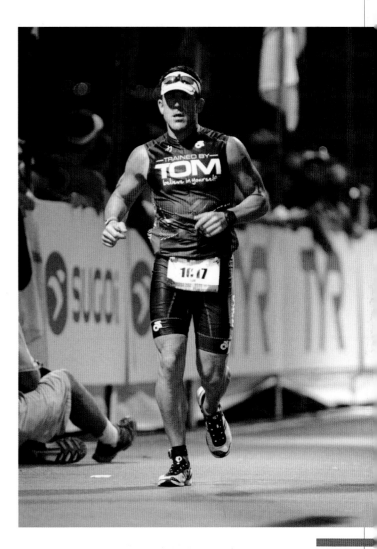

The author at the finish line of the Hawaii Ironman World Championships

# PART 4

## Recipes for
## Triathletes

# Power Meals and Power Smoothies

**HERE ARE FORTY-FIVE HEALTHY, YET** simple meal options and ten smoothies to fuel your triathlon lifestyle. They are broken down by breakfast, lunch, and dinner, but you can have any of these meals at any time of the day, depending on your needs and what you are hungry for. I love eating meals that are traditionally considered as dinners for breakfast and breakfast meals for dinner. The choice is yours.

These meals are also broken down into three categories based on their calorie count: 400 to 500 calories, 500 to 600 calories, and a hefty 600 to 700 calories. This gives you even more options based on your personal nutritional needs, which can vary day to day and even meal to meal based on your weight, workout load, and more.

For those times when you don't feel like eating or are pressed for time, and a shake is an easier way to quickly take in your carbohydrates and protein, there are an additional ten power smoothies to choose from. These range in calories from several hundred all the way up to whopping 800

to 900 calorie concoctions. Just finished a brutal brick workout, a 100-mile (161 km) bike ride, followed by a thirty-minute run in preparation for your upcoming Ironman? A 900-calorie beast of a power smoothie might just be the recovery meal you need.

As I have said throughout the book, success comes down to doing the little things consistently, and this is especially true when it comes to what we eat each and every day. Take the time to shop intelligently and stock your kitchen with a wide assortment of healthy foods. Take the little extra time it takes to prepare your own healthy meals whenever possible. I am the last person who wants to spend a significant amount of time in the kitchen preparing something that will take me but a few minutes to eat. Food is fuel to me, so these recipes are extremely simple to prepare. They will in fact make a huge positive impact on how you feel, how you look, and ultimately how you perform on race day, so the small investment of time will reap huge rewards.

# Breakfast

## The Bowl

- ½ cup (40 g) oats (measured dry)
- Mix in 1½ tablespoons (24 g) peanut butter OR 2 tablespoons (18 g) chopped nuts
- 6 ounces (170 g) low-fat Greek yogurt
- 1 fruit OR ¼ cup (35 g) dried fruit in oatmeal

## The Breakfast Sandwich

- 1 whole wheat English muffin OR 2 slices double-fiber bread
- 2 to 3 ounces (56.7 to 85 g) lean Canadian bacon/ham/turkey sausage
- 1 slice 2 percent cheese
- 1 egg
- 1 fruit

## The Basic Breakfast

- 1 egg and 2 egg whites
- 2 slices turkey bacon
- 2 slices whole wheat toast with thin spread butter and cinnamon
- 6 ounces (170 g) low-fat Greek yogurt

## The Parfait

- 6 ounces (170 g) low-fat Greek yogurt
- 1 tablespoon (20 g) honey and 1 cup (145 g) berries mixed in yogurt
- ¼ cup (20 g) low-fat granola
- 2 eggs

## On-the-Go Breakfast

- 200-calorie energy bar
- 1 string cheese
- 1 banana
- 10 to 15 almonds

# Lunch

## Mix-n-Match

- 15 whole wheat crackers
- 2 ounces (56.7 g) lean deli meat
- One 2 percent string cheese
- 6 ounces (170 g) low-fat Greek yogurt with ½ cup (72.5 g) berries and ½ a banana

## Pack the Pita

- 1 whole wheat pita with 2 to 3 ounces (56.7 to 85 g) chicken breast, ¼ cup (30 g) 2 percent grated cheese, veggies, ⅓ of an avocado
- Side salad with dressing on the side
- 1 fruit

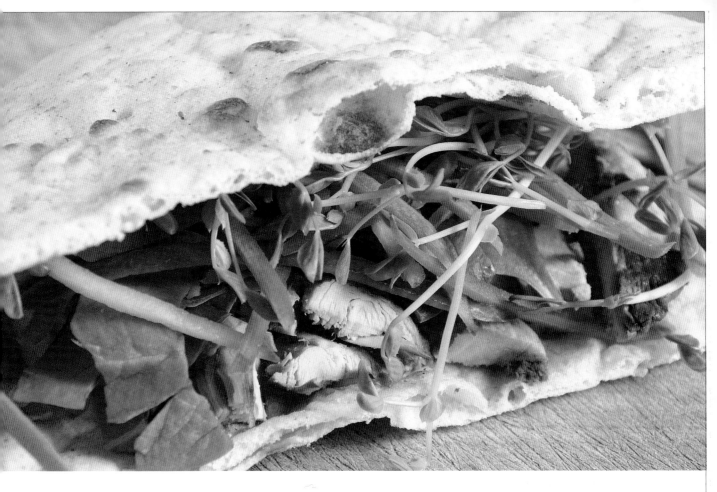

## Old School

- Peanut butter and jelly sandwich on whole wheat bread (2 tablespoons [32 g] peanut butter and 1 tablespoon [20 g] jelly)
- 1 fruit

## Go Fish

- 3 ounces (85 g) albacore tuna in water with 1 tablespoon (14 g) light mayo and some mustard, veggies of choice, and 1 tablespoon (7 g) chopped pecans
- 2 slices whole wheat bread **OR** 15 whole wheat crackers
- 1 small fruit **OR** ½ cup (75 g) chopped fruit

## Wrap It Up

- 1 whole wheat tortilla
- 3 ounces (85 g) grilled chicken breast
- Veggies
- 1 slice 2 percent cheese **OR** ¼ cup (30 g) grated 2 percent cheese
- 1 to 2 tablespoons (15 to 30 g) hummus
- 10 whole wheat crackers
- Salad with dressing on the side

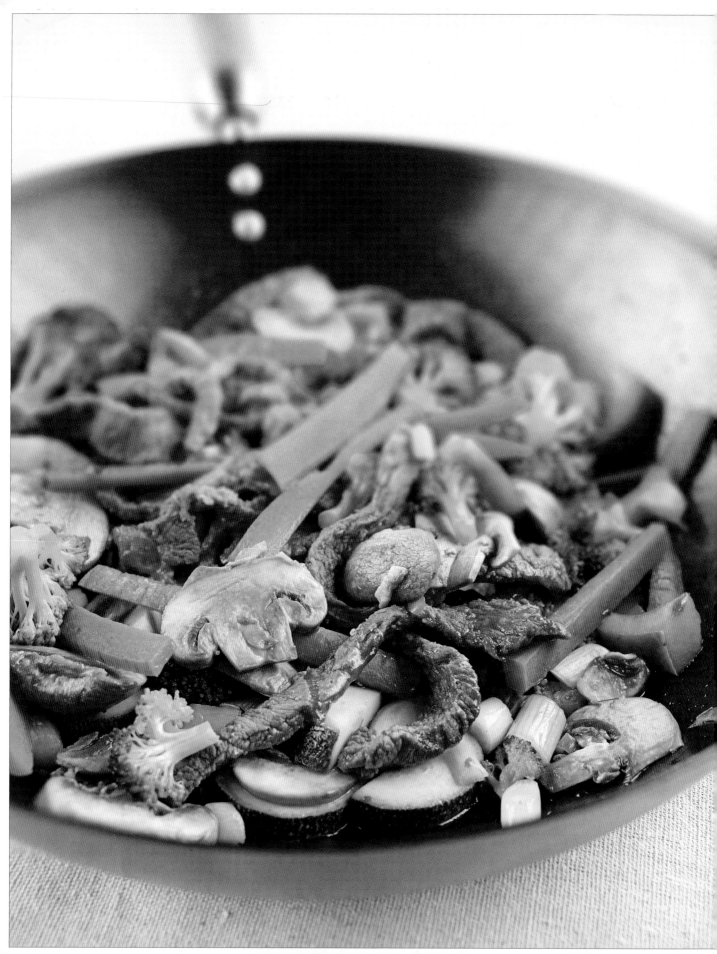

# Dinner

## The Basic

- 4 ounces (113.4 g) meat (palm-size) (chicken, fish, beef, pork, or turkey)
- 1 to 2 cups (200 to 400 g) vegetables
- 1 cup (140 g) carbohydrate (pasta, rice, potato, sweet potato, quinoa, couscous, corn, fruit, or bread)
- Side salad with dressing on the side

## Stir-Fry

- 4 ounces (113.4 g) grilled chicken breast
- 2 to 3 cups (400 to 600 g) vegetables, sautéed
- 1 cup (195 g) cooked brown rice
- Soy sauce, to taste

  *Mix all items together.

## Taco Salad

- 3 to 5 cups (165 to 275 g) lettuce and veggies
- ¼ cup (30 g) 2 percent grated cheese
- 1 cup (225 g) ground turkey meat browned on stove with taco seasoning
- ¼ cup (41 g) yellow corn OR (43 g) black beans
- ½ cup (112.5 g) guacamole
- 8 light tortilla chips, crumbled
- Salsa, to taste

## Pita Pizza

- 1 whole wheat pita
- ¼ cup (61 g) tomato sauce
- ⅓ cup (40 g) 2 percent grated cheese
- Cover with 2 to 3 ounces (56.7 to 85 g) cooked chicken OR turkey OR turkey sausage

  *Broil in the oven for 4 to 5 minutes.
- Salad with 2 tablespoons (18 g) dried fruit, 2 tablespoons (18 g) nuts, and dressing on the side

## Burger Bash

- 100 percent whole grain hamburger bun
- 4 ounces (113.4 g) lean ground meat patty
- Veggies
- 1 to 2 tablespoons (9 to 18 g) smashed avocado
- Big salad with lots of veggies, 2 tablespoons (18 g) nuts, and dressing on the side

---

**MEAL OPTIONS:
500 TO 600 CALORIES**

---

# Breakfast

## Waffle Iron

- 2 whole wheat waffles
- 1 tablespoon (16 g) peanut butter spread on each waffle (can add cinnamon)
- 8 ounces (236.6 ml) low-fat milk with ½ scoop whey protein powder

### Bacon, Egg, and Cheese Sandwich

- 1 whole wheat English muffin
- 3 ounces (56.7 g) lean Canadian bacon
- 1 slice 2 percent cheese
- 1 egg
- 4 ounces (113.4 g) low-fat Greek yogurt with ¼ cup (20 g) low-fat granola

### This-n-That

- 1 egg and 2 whites and veggies
- 1 slice whole wheat toast with 1 tablespoon (16 g) peanut butter
- ½ cup (75 g) berries
- 8 ounces (236.6 ml) low-fat milk with ½ scoop protein powder

### Smoothie

- 1 scoop whey protein
- 4 ounces (113.4 g) low-fat vanilla Greek yogurt
- 8 ounces (236.6 ml) low-fat milk
- 1 banana
- ½ cup (75 g) berries
- 1 tablespoon (16 g) almond butter

### Cereal Combo

- 2 eggs with veggies
- 1¼ cups (120 g) whole grain cereal with low-fat milk
- 1 banana
- 8 ounces (236.6 ml) low-fat milk

# Lunch

### Flatout

- High-protein wrap, such as Flatout
- ⅓ cup (40 g) grated 2 percent cheese
- 3 to 4 ounces (85 to 113.4 g) lean meat
- Veggies
- 1 tablespoon (15 g) light sauce
- 1 cup (145 g) strawberries and 8 to 10 grapes
- 15 whole wheat crackers OR pretzels

### Taco Tuesday

- Two 6-inch (15.2 cm) white corn tortillas, each stuffed with:
  - 2 ounces (56.7 g) grilled Mahi Mahi
  - 1 to 2 tablespoons (7.5 to 15 g) Mexican Cheese
  - ¼ cup (43 g) black beans
  - ¼ avocado
- Salad with ¼ cup (41 g) corn, tomato, red peppers, and dressing on the side

### Brown Bag

- Sandwich on whole wheat bread with:
  - 1 slice 2 percent cheese
  - 4 ounces (113.4 g) lean meat
  - Veggies
  - 2 tablespoons (31 g) hummus
- 10 whole wheat crackers OR pretzels
- 1 cup (150 g) chopped fruit OR a banana

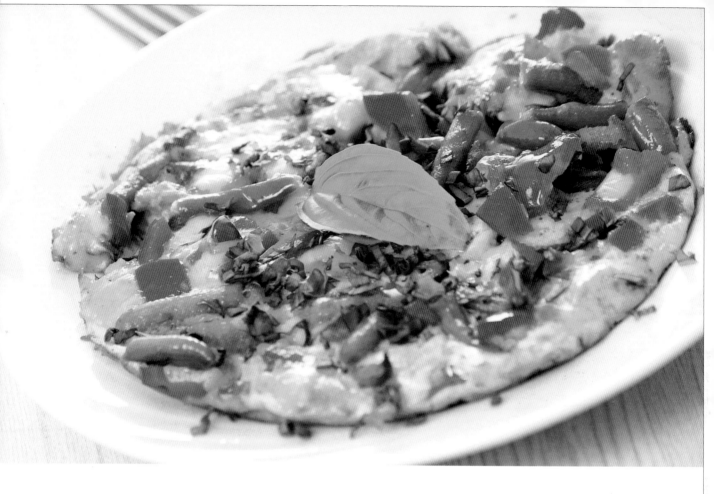

## Warm Salmon Salad

- ½ bag 90-Second Multi-Grain Rice Pilaf
- 4 to 5 ounces (113.4 to 141.8 g) grilled salmon
- 2 cups (60 g) sautéed spinach (lightly with olive oil)

## The Snack Baggie

- ½ peanut butter and jelly sandwich with 1 tablespoon (16 g) peanut butter and 1 tablespoon (20 g) jelly
- 10 whole wheat crackers **OR** pretzels
- 6 ounces (170 g) low-fat Greek yogurt with ¼ cup (20 g) granola and ½ cup (75 g) chopped fruit
- 1 string cheese

# Dinner

## The Basic

- 5 ounces (141.8 g) meat (hand-size) (chicken, fish, beef, pork, or turkey)
- 1 to 2 cups (200 to 400 g) vegetables
- 1¼ cups (175 g) carbohydrates (pasta, rice, potato, sweet potato, quinoa, couscous, corn, fruit, or bread)
- Side salad with dressing on the side

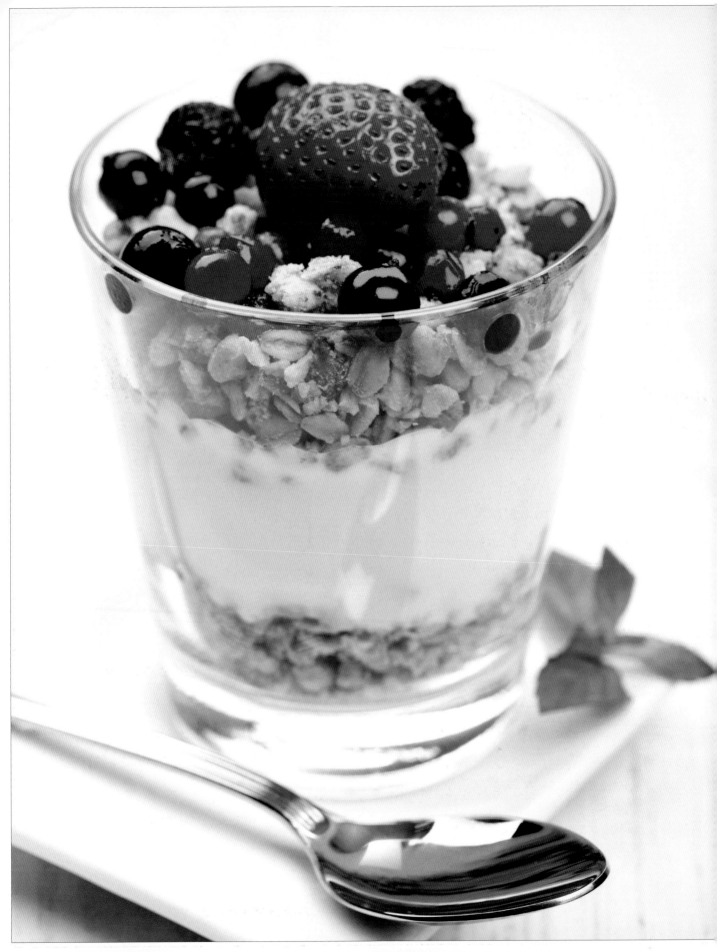

## Go Green

- Large salad with mixed greens and veggies
- 5 ounces (141.8 g) grilled chicken breast
- 3 tablespoons (27 g) nuts
- ½ cup (75 g) chopped berries
- Dressing on the side
- 1 large sweet potato baked with skin, drizzled with olive oil

## Chicken Parmesan

- 5 ounces (141.8 g) chicken breast breaded with egg white, Italian-seasoned bread crumbs, and 2 tablespoons (10 g) reduced-fat Parmesan cheese
- 1¼ cup (175 g) al dente spinach pasta cooked and topped with ½ cup (123 g) Healthy Choice tomato sauce
- 1 cup (30 g) fresh spinach mixed in with pasta
- 2 cups (400 g) Italian vegetables (veggies of choice baked in oven with Italian seasoning)

## The Shroom

- 2 portobello mushrooms grilled, each stuffed with:
  - 2½ ounces (70.9 g) chopped, cooked chicken
  - Veggies of choice (cooked lightly in extra-virgin olive oil)
  - ¾ cup (146 g) cooked brown OR whole grain rice pilaf
- Salad with veggies and dressing on the side

## Healthy Quesadilla

- 1 whole wheat tortilla
- ½ cup (60 g) 2 percent grated cheese
- 5 ounces (141.8 g) chopped chicken breast
  *Fold over and broil in the oven 2 minutes per side.
- ⅓ of an avocado
- 10 light tortilla chips and salsa
- Side salad with dressing on the side

**MEAL OPTIONS:
600 TO 700 CALORIES**

# Breakfast

## Clean Breakfast

- 2 cups (300 g) fruit
- 1 egg
- 1 cup (225 g) low-fat cottage cheese
- 15 to 20 almonds

## The Real Bacon Deal

- 2 eggs with sprinkle of 2 percent grated cheese
- 3 to 4 slices bacon
- 2 slices whole wheat toast with 1 tablespoon (20 g) 100 percent fruit jelly on each slice toast
- 1 fruit
- 8 ounces (236.6 ml) low-fat milk

### Oats and More

- 1 cup (80 g) steel-cut oats, mixed with:
  - 1 tablespoon (20 g) honey
  - ¼ cup (38 g) fruit
  - 1½ (24 g) tablespoons natural peanut butter
- 1 egg and 3 egg whites

### Smoothie Satisfaction

- 1 scoop whey protein
- 8 ounces (236.6 ml) low-fat milk
- 4 ounces (113.4 g) low-fat Greek yogurt
- 1 cup (145 g) berries
- 2 tablespoons (40 g) honey
- 2 tablespoons (10 g) dry oats
- 1 tablespoon (16 g) peanut butter

### Quick Bites

- 5–6 peanut butter balls made with:
  - ½ cup (130 g) peanut butter
  - ¼ cup (80 g) honey
  - 1 cup (80 g) oats
  - ½ cup (64 g) whey protein powder

  *Mix the peanut butter and honey together. Then stir in the oats and protein powder. Roll into 22 balls and refrigerate.
- 1 banana
- 16 ounces (473.2 ml) low-fat milk

# Lunch

### Roll-Ups

- 5 to 6 (141.8 to 170 g) ounces lean deli meat
- 2 ounces (56.7 g) 2 percent cheese
- All sorts of veggies

  *Roll meat, cheese and veggies into two 6-inch (15.2 cm) whole wheat tortillas.
- 1 fruit

### The Basic Bigger Lunch

- Sandwich on whole wheat bread with:
  - 1 slice 2 percent Swiss cheese
  - 6 ounces (170 g) smoked turkey
  - Veggies
  - Drizzled pesto
- 15 whole wheat crackers **OR** pretzels
- 1 fruit
- 10 almonds

### Grilled Cheese

- 2 slices whole wheat bread toasted in pan with:
  - 1 to 2 tablespoons (14 to 28 g) yogurt-based butter
  - 2 slices 2 percent cheese
  - 3 ounces (85 g) lean ham
- 150- to 200-calorie serving of tomato soup

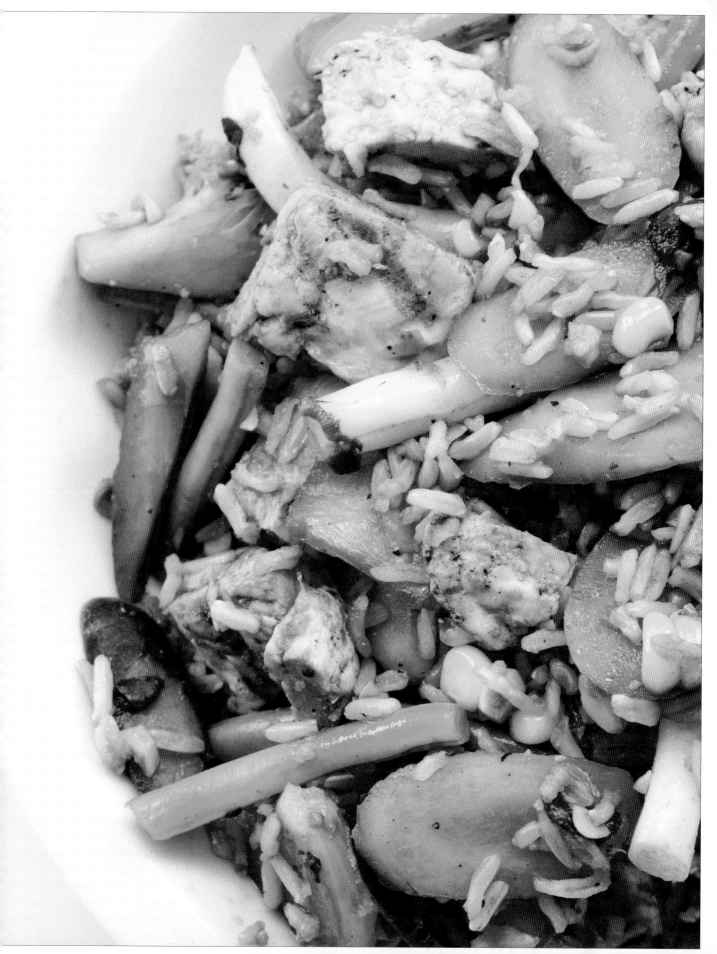

### Twisted Philly Cheese Bagel

- 1 whole wheat bagel
- 4 ounces (113.4 g) lean roast beef
- 1 slice 2 percent Provolone cheese
- 1 apple sliced, covered in cinnamon and microwaved until soft and then drizzled with 4 ounces (113.4 g) low-fat Greek yogurt

### Tuna Melt

- 2 whole wheat English muffins toasted, each with:
  - 2 ounces (56.7 g) tuna (canned in water)
  - 1 slice 2 percent Swiss cheese (melted)
- Veggies of choice
- ½ to 1 cup (75 to 150 g) chopped fruit

# Dinner

### Simple Dinner

- 7 ounces (198.5 g) meat (chicken, fish, beef, pork, or turkey)
- 2 cups (400 g) vegetables drizzled with extra-virgin olive oil
- ½ cup (210 g) carbohydrates (rice, pasta, potato, quinoa, fruit, beans, corn, or bread)
- Side salad with dressing on the side

### Go Lean

- Big salad with 7 ounces (198.5 g) grilled chicken breast, 3 tablespoons (27 g) nuts and ½ cup (95 g) mandarin oranges
- 1 large fruit OR 1¼ cup (45 g) chopped
- 2 slices whole wheat bread/toast OR 15 whole wheat crackers

### Lettuce Wraps

- 7 ounces (198.5 g) diced chicken cooked with water chestnuts, chives, and vegetables of choice
- Soy sauce to taste
- Large iceberg lettuce leaves
  *Roll the filling into the lettuce leaves.
- 1½ cups (293 g) cooked brown rice

### Breakfast for Dinner

- 2 whole wheat tortillas, each with:
  - 1 egg and 3 egg whites
  - ¼ cup (30 g) 2 percent cheese and veggies
- 1 fruit

### Salmon Sliders

- 3 mini slider buns (whole wheat if possible), each with:
  - 2 ounces (56.7 g) salmon
  - Spinach and a slice of tomato
  - Grilled onions
  - 1 teaspoon (5 g) pesto mayo
- Mixed green salad with dressing on the side

# 300-Calorie Smoothies

## Basic Berry Smoothie

- 1 cup (236.6 ml) 2 percent milk
- 1 scoop whey protein powder
- 1 cup (145 g) berries

## Chocolate Banana Smoothie

- ½ cup (118.3 ml) 2 percent milk
- 6 ounces (170 g) low-fat Greek yogurt
- 1 banana
- 1 to 2 tablespoons (20 to 40 g) chocolate syrup

# 500-Calorie Smoothies

## Nutter Butter Smoothie

- 1 cup (236.6 ml) 2 percent milk
- 1 scoop whey protein powder
- 1 banana
- 1 tablespoon (20 g) honey
- 1 tablespoon (16 g) peanut butter

## Hot Chocolate Smoothie

- 1 cup (236.6 ml) 2 percent milk
- 1 scoop whey protein powder
- 1 banana
- 2 packets hot chocolate (can be sugar-free)

## Two-Ingredient Smoothie

- 2 cups (473.2 ml) 2 percent milk
- 2 scoops high-calorie protein powder

## Peanut Butter Banana Smoothie

- 1 cup (236.6 ml) 2 percent milk
- 1 scoop high-calorie protein powder
- 1 banana
- 1 tablespoon (16 g) peanut butter

# 700-Calorie Smoothies

## High-Cal Honey Smoothie

- 1½ cups (354.9 ml) 2 percent milk
- 3 scoops high-calorie protein powder
- 1 tablespoon (20 g) honey

## Berry Flax Smoothie

- 2 cups (473.2 ml) 2 percent milk
- 2 scoops high-calorie protein powder
- 1 tablespoon (28 ml) flax seed oil
- 1 cup (145 g) berries

# 800 to 1,000-Calorie Smoothies

## Berry Booster Smoothie

- 2 cups (473.2 ml) 2 percent milk
- 3 to 4 scoops high-calorie protein powder
- 1 cup (145 g) berries

## Seedy Banana Smoothie

- 2 cups (473.2 ml) 2 percent milk
- 3 scoops high-calorie protein powder
- 2 tablespoons (26 g) chia seeds
- 1 cup (145 g) berries

## SMOOTHIE-MAKING TIPS

- If you're looking to reduce calories, you can opt for skim (fat-free) milk.

- If you're trying to get extra calories (as in the high-calorie shakes), add a high-calorie protein powder that includes carbohydrate and protein because those contain more calories than whey isolate protein powder.

- If you're lactose intolerant, you can substitute Lactaid milk for regular milk for an exact protein and nutrient exchange minus the lactose.

- If you have a milk allergy, you can sub out milk for soy milk for similar protein and calories. However, milks such as rice, almond, and coconut do not provide the same protein as regular milk, so you need to add more protein powder (soy, hemp, pea, egg white, etc.) to get in adequate protein.

- If you are not a vegetable lover, you can experiment with mixing spinach into the smoothies with fruit.

- If you would like to get more carbohydrate and a little less protein in your smoothie, you can sub 100 percent fruit juice for milk.

- Add ice to your liking.

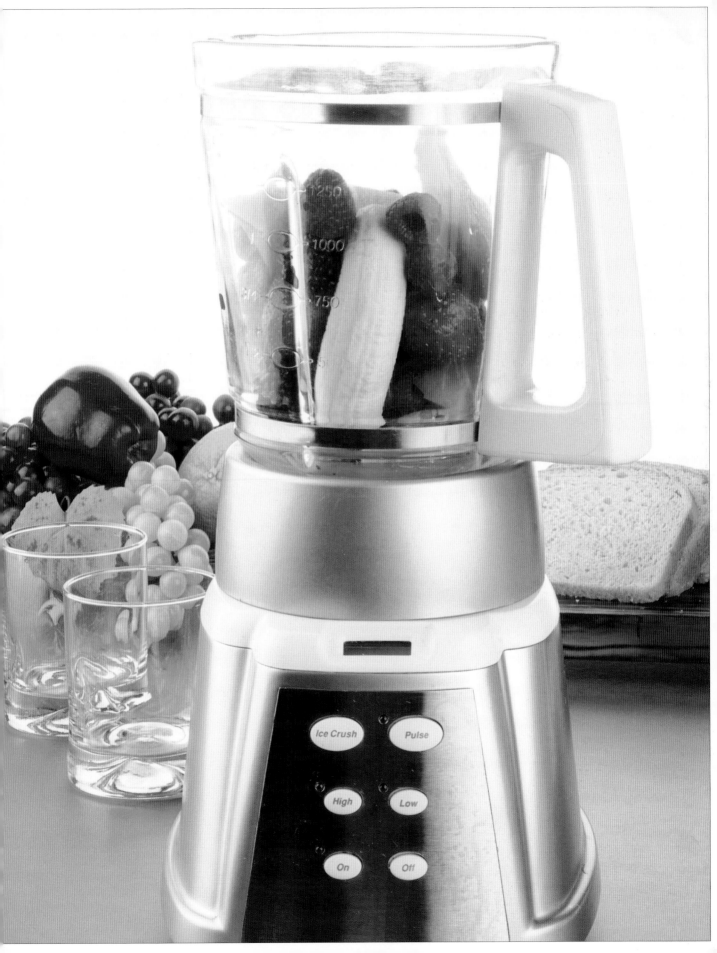

# Resources

American College of Sports Medicine. *ACSM's Guidelines for Exercise Testing and Prescription*, 9th edition. (Philadelphia: Lippincott Williams & Wilkins, 2013.)

American Council on Exercise. *Ace Lifestyle & Weight Management Consultant Manual: The Ultimate Resource for Fitness Professionals*. (San Diego: American Council on Exercise, 2009.)

Antonio, J., et al. (eds.). *Essentials of Sports Nutrition and Supplements*. (New York: Humana Press, 2008.)

Benardot, D. *Advanced Sports Nutrition*, 2nd edition. (Champaign: Human Kinetics, 2011.)

Bryant, C. X., and D. J. Green. (Eds.). *ACE Personal Trainer Manual: The Ultimate Resource for Fitness Professionals*, 3rd edition. (Monterey: Healthy Learning, 2003.)

Clark, N. Nancy *Clark's Sports Nutrition Guidebook*, 5th Edition. (Champaign: Human Kinetics, 2013.)

Howley, E. T., and B. D. Franks. *Health Fitness Instructor's Handbook*, 3rd edition. (Champaign: Human Kinetics, 1997.)

McGinnis, P. M. *Biomechanics of Sport and Exercise*. (Champaign: Human Kinetics, 2004.)

Powers, S., and E. Howley. *Exercise Physiology: Theory and Application to Fitness and Performance*, 8th Edition. (New York: McGraw-Hill Humanities/Social Sciences/Languages, 2011.)

Wilmore, J. H, D. Costill, and W. L. Kenney. *Physiology of Sport and Exercise*, 4th Edition. (Champaign: Human Kinetics, 2007.)

# Acknowledgments

First and foremost I would like to thank my incredible wife Philippa; without her support, nothing I do would be possible.

I would also like to thank my amazing literary agent, Lauren Galit of the LKG Agency, for putting up with me; my editor Jessica Haberman for her unending patience and guidance; and Amy Goodson for lending her wealth of expertise and her fantastic recipes.

Finally, I would like to thank my two boys, Tommy and Cooper, for giving me the ultimate motivation to be the healthiest role model possible.

**—TOM**

First, I would like to thank Tom Holland for giving me the opportunity to add to and be a part of this great book! I would also like to thank Linda Melone for introducing to me to Tom and starting me down this journey. Finally, to all of my clients who are swimming, biking and running daily... you are an inspiration! This is for you!

**—AMY**

# About the Authors

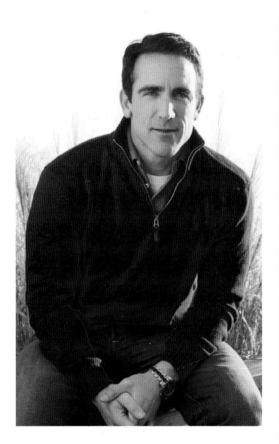

**TOM HOLLAND,** author of *The 12-Week Triathlete* and *Marathon Method* (both Fair Winds Press) and *Beat the Gym* (Harper-Collins), is an exercise physiologist and certified sports nutritionist who has coached thousands of people to reach their fitness goals; from losing weight to climbing mountains, running marathons, and completing Ironman triathlons. Tom is a Certified Strength and Conditioning Specialist certified by the National Strength and Conditioning Association (NSCA-CSCS) and has also been certified by the American College of Sports Medicine (ACSM), the American Council on Exercise (ACE), the National Academy of Sports Medicine (NASM), and the Aerobics and Fitness Association of America (AFAA). He began as a personal trainer and fitness instructor in New York City, working at such facilities as the Reebok Sports Club, Equinox, Crunch, The New York Sports Clubs, and the Cardio Fitness Center. He then struck out on his own, founding TeamHolland LLC and expanding into new areas of the fitness industry. Tom has run more than 60 marathons and ultra marathons and won the 2007 Dutchess County Classic marathon. He is a 21-time Ironman triathlete in races around the world. He is head coach of the Multiple Myeloma Research Foundation's Power Team and created the triathlon program for the SmileTrain charity. He has appeared as a fitness expert on NBC, CNN Headline News, and ABC's Good Morning America.

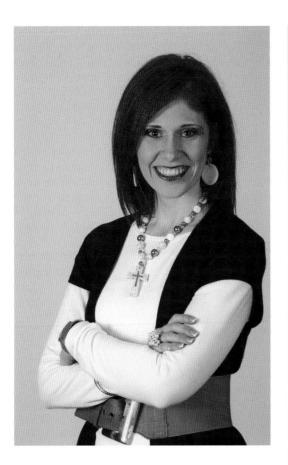

**AMY GOODSON,** M.S., R.D., C.S.S.D., L.D., is a registered dietitian in the Dallas/Fort Worth metroplex. She received her bachelor of science degree in speech communications from Texas Christian University and a masters degree in exercise and sports nutrition from Texas Woman's University.

Currently, Amy is the full-time sports dietitian for Ben Hogan Sports Medicine, where she works with athletes of all levels, serves as a media dietitian, and speaks to sports teams as well as at a variety of nutrition, athletic training, and coaching conferences. Amy is the sports dietitian for Texas Christian University Athletics, University of Texas at Arlington Athletics, and is the consulting sports R.D. for the Dallas Cowboys, Texas Rangers, FC Dallas soccer team, and Jim McLean Golf School where she works with amateur and professional golfers. In addition, she is an adjunct professor and dietetic intern preceptor for Texas Woman's University, Texas Christian University, and the University of Texas at Arlington and is a state media representative for the Texas Academy of Nutrition and Dietetics.

# Index

"80/20 Rule," 8, 85, 107

## A

aid stations, 117, 120–121, 139, 149–150
alcohol, 84–85, 102
all-natural diet, 112–113
amino acids, 37–38, 66–67
appetite increase, 24–25
Atkins diet, 112

## B

Bacon, Egg, and Cheese Sandwich, 174
The Basic (dinner recipes), 173, 175
The Basic Bigger Lunch, 178
The Basic Breakfast, 170
bathroom breaks, 59
Bento Box, 118, 120
Berry Smoothies, 181–182
bike
    excess weight on, 116–117
    fueling on the, 128–129, 138–139, 147–148,
      162–165
    gear considerations, 157–158
Body Mass Index (BMI), 81
"bonking," 29–33, 76, 138, 153, 164
The Bowl (breakfast recipe), 170
branched chain amino acids (BCAA), 66–67
Brazier, Brendan, 107
breakfast examples, pre-race, 127, 136, 147, 161
Breakfast for Dinner, 180
breakfast recipes, 170, 173–174, 177–178
The Breakfast Sandwich, 170
Brown Bag (lunch recipe), 174
Burger Bash, 173

## C

caffeine, as ergogenic aid, 57, 70–71, 161, 166
calorie-based meal options
    400-500 calories, 170–173
    500-600 calories, 173–177
    600-700 calories, 177–180
    Smoothies, 174, 178, 181–182
calories
    about, 22–24
    body storage of, 29, 125, 134, 155
    recovery/refueling and, 100–101
    weight loss and, 50–51, 83–85, 97–98, 106
carbohydrates
    glycemic index and, 35
    good vs. bad, 33–34
    in recovery products, 64
    simple vs. complex, 102
    in sports drinks, 58
    as supplement, 67
    types of, 27–29
    and the wall, 29–30
carbo-loading, 134–135, 142–143, 155–156
celiac disease, 111
"Central Governor Theory," 30
Cereal Combo, 174
chia seeds, 65
Chicken Parmesan, 177
Chocolate Banana Smoothie, 181
chocolate milk, 103
cholesterol, 47
chondroitin sulfate, 66
Clean Breakfast, 177
compensatory eating, 24–25, 98
cramping, muscle, 68–69, 112, 148–150, 156,
  164–166

## D

destination races, planning for, 159
Dietary Supplement Health and Education Act
  (DSHEA), 62
diets
  about, 105–106, 113
  all-natural, 112–113
  Atkins, 112
  fad, 78, 105, 111
  flexitarian, 108
  gluten-free, 111–112
  lacto-ovo vegetarian, 108–109
  macrobiotic, 110
  Paleo, 111
  pescetarian, 108
  raw food, 109–110
  vegan, 40, 109–110
  vegetarian, 38, 40, 107–108
  The Zone, 112
dinner examples, pre-race, 146, 158–160
dinner recipes, 173, 175, 177, 180
disaccharides, 28
diuretic effect, 70
DNF (Did Not Finish), 20, 29

## E

electrolytes, 58–59, 67–70, 100
ergogenic aids, 57, 62, 161

## F

fad diets, 78, 105, 111
fatigue, minimizing, 25, 29, 54–55, 70–71, 150
fat(s)
  bad, 40, 47–48

body, 77–81
burning, 50–51, 70–71, 90–91
calories in, 39, 45
good, 48–50, 65
recovery products and, 64
storage process of, 46
fiber, 28, 33–35, 111
Flatout (lunch recipe), 174
flexitarian diet, 108
Food and Drug Administration (FDA), 62
food journals, 83, 93–94
FRS sports nutrition, 38, 103
fructose, 28, 34, 143
fuel belts, 121–122, 164–165
fueling
  deliberate under-, 90–91
  experimenting with, 87–88
  inadequate, 25, 30–33, 89
  See also recovery/refueling

## G

gastrointestinal distress
  caffeine and, 71
  pre-race jitters and, 125–127, 130
  sports drinks and, 58, 68, 88, 143, 165
  working through, 165
Gatorade, 58–59, 112
  See also sports drinks
gear bags, for Ironman triathlon, 157–158
gels, 67, 92
glucosamine/chondroitin, 66
glucose, 27–28, 35
gluten-free diet, 111–112
glycemic index (GI), 35
On-the-Go Breakfast, 170

Go Fish (lunch recipe), 171
Go Green (dinner recipe), 177
Go Lean (dinner recipe), 180
Grilled Cheese, 178
GU, 67

## H

half Ironman distance triathlons, 141–150
HDL cholesterol, 47–49
Healthy Quesadilla, 177
High-Cal Honey Smoothie, 181
Hot Chocolate Smoothie, 181
hunger. See appetite increase
hydration
    about, 53
    bathroom breaks and, 59
    daily, 54
    race day, 127, 135–139, 144–146, 156–157
    water vs. sports drinks, 57–58
    workout, 55–56, 89–90
hydrogenation, 47
hyponatremia, 56–57

## I

inflammation, muscle, 50, 65
Ironman distance triathlons
    about, 153–154
    bike/gear considerations, 157–158
    post-race fueling for, 166–167
    pre-race fueling for, 155–161

## J

jitters, pre-race, 125–127, 160
joint pain, reducing, 50, 65–66
junk food, 23–24, 84
Jurek, Scott, 107

## L

lacto-ovo vegetarian diet, 108–109

lactose, 28, 34, 182
LaLanne, Jack, 34
LDL cholesterol, 40, 47–48
Lettuce Wraps, 180
lunch recipes, 170–171, 174–175, 178, 180

## M

macrobiotic diet, 110
macronutrients
    carbohydrates, 27–35
    diets and, 106, 112–113
    fats, 45–51
    protein, 37–43
Manhattan to Montauk bike ride, 30–33
metabolic window, 34, 64, 98, 100
metabolism, 39, 43, 78, 105
Mix-n-Match (lunch recipe), 170
monosaccharides, 27–28
monounsaturated fats, 48–49
multivitamins, 64–65
muscle(s)
    cramping, 68–69, 112, 148–150, 156, 164–166
    inflammation, 50, 65
    loss, 23, 43
    metabolic window and, 34
    protein and, 37–39, 42–43
    weight, 80–81

## N

nutrition plans, importance of, 12–13, 19–20, 82–83
Nutter Butter Smoothie, 181

## O

Oats and More, 178
Old School (lunch recipe), 171
Olympic distance triathlons, 133–139
omega-3/6 fats, 49–50, 65
osteoarthritis, 66

## P

Pack the Pita, 170

Paleo diet, 111

The Parfait, 170

peanut butter, 83–84

Peanut Butter Balls, 146, 178

Peanut Butter Banana Smoothie, 181

peeing, on the bike, 59

pescetarian diet, 108

Pita Pizza, 173

placebo effect, 71–72

polysaccharides, 28

polyunsaturated fats, 49–50

post-workout fueling. See recovery/refueling

potassium, 68–69

Powerade, 58

   See also sports drinks

pre-workout fueling

   carbohydrates and, 67

   glycemic index and, 35

   hydration and, 59

   options for, 89–93, 102

   for race day, 125–128, 131, 135–136, 142–147, 154–162

   and the wall, 29–33

protein

   excess, 40

   metabolic window and, 34, 100–101

   muscle and, 37–39, 42–43

   plant-based, 109

   powders/shakes, 38, 63–64, 82

   requirements, 39

   sources of, 40–43, 108–109

## Q

Quesadilla, Healthy, 177

Quick Bites, 146, 178

## R

race-day fueling

   half Ironman distance, 141–150

   Ironman distance, 153–167

   logistics of, 115–122

   Olympic distance, 133–139

   sprint distance, 125–131

raw food diet, 109–110

The Real Bacon Deal, 177

recipes

   breakfast, 170, 173–174, 177–178

   dinner, 173, 175, 177, 180

   lunch, 170–171, 174–175, 178, 180

   smoothies, 174, 178, 181–182

recovery/refueling, 24–25, 34, 64, 97–103, 139, 150, 166–167

Roll, Rich, 107

Roll-Ups, 178

run, fueling your, 92, 94, 120–121, 139, 149–150, 165–166

## S

Salmon Sliders, 180

salt supplementation, 68–70, 145, 148, 150, 156

salty sweater, 57–58

sarcopenia, 43

saturated fat, 47–48

Sears, Barry, 112

Seedy Banana Smoothie, 182

The Shroom, 177

Simple Dinner, 180

Smoothie recipes, 174, 178, 181–182

The Snack Baggie (lunch recipe), 175

sodium. See salt supplementation

special needs bags, Ironman triathlon, 158

sports drinks

   all-natural diet and, 112

   gastrointestinal distress and, 58, 68, 88, 143, 165

   pre-workout fueling, 90, 92

on race day, 128–129, 135–138, 145–150, 156–157, 161–167

as supplement, 67–69

vs. water, 57–58

sprint triathlons, 125–131

Stir-Fry, 173

strength training, 81

sucrose, 28

supermarket tips, 48

supplements

about, 61–63

for daily life and training, 63–71

placebo effect and, 71–72

vs. real food, 103

sweat rate, 57

## T

T1 (transition 1), 115–116, 128, 137, 147, 157, 162

T2 (transition 2), 115–116, 129–130, 139, 148–149, 157–158, 164

Taco Salad, 173

Taco Tuesday, 174

thirst, 55

This-n-That (breakfast recipe), 174

trans fat, 47–48

Tuna Melt, 180

Twisted Philly Cheese Bagel, 180

Two-Ingredient Smoothie, 181

## U

unsaturated fats, 48–50

urinating, on the bike, 59

urine color, 54, 135, 156

## V

vegan diet, 40, 109–110

vegetarian diet, 38, 40, 107–108

VO2 max, 80

## W

WADA (World Anti-Doping Agency), 70

Waffle Iron, 173

wall, hitting the, 29–33, 76, 153, 164

Warm Salmon Salad, 175

water. See hydration

water bottles

on the bike, 116–118, 120

on the run, 121

weight

bike, 116–117

gain, 24–25, 57

loss, 23, 50–51, 75–85, 97–98, 106

workouts, fueling, 87–94

World Anti-Doping Agency (WADA), 70

World Triathlon Corporation, 165

## Z

The Zone Diet, 112